AIDS

AIDS

Meeting
the
community
challenge

edited by
Vicky Cosstick

Preface by
Cardinal Basil Hume

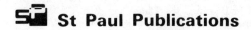 **St Paul Publications**

The Publishers are grateful to Times Newspapers Ltd, for permission to reproduce "Time for a moral renaissance" by Cardinal Basil Hume and "Only a moral revolution can contain this scourge" by Sir Immanuel Jakobowits, and to *The Tablet*, where "Aids and morality" by Dr Jack Dominian and parts of "Aids and sex education" by Justin Price OSB previously appeared.

Cover design: Mary Lou Winters

St Paul Publications
Middlegreen, Slough SL3 6BT, England

Copyright © St Paul Publications 1987

Photoset by Grove Graphics, Tring
Printed by Billing & Sons, Worcester

ISBN 085439 264 5

St Paul Publications is an activity of the priests and brothers of the Society of St Paul and the Daughters of St Paul who proclaim the Gospel through the media of social communication

CONTENTS

PART VII: THE CHRISTIAN AND THE SECULAR

PREFACE

Cardinal Basil Hume

Einstein once said that the unleashed power of the atom had changed everything except our ways of thinking. The same may be true in human relationships after the outbreak of Aids. We come to terms with radical change only with the greatest reluctance and often too late. While there is some panic over the new threat to health, much current sexual behaviour remains unchanged. The moral landscape has in fact altered irrevocably with the onset of Aids. Even the merciful discovery of an antidote should not be hailed as heralding an automatic return to ways of behaving and moral attitudes now dramatically discredited. We need a more fundamental reappraisal.

The Church has an indispensable role to play. It must be unyielding in principle and compassionate in practice. The Church must clearly condemn sin but never disown the sinner. The Gospel account of the woman taken in adultery provides the best indication of the Christian attitude. No onlooker is to cast the first stone but the woman herself is told to sin no more. A word of caution is necessary from the outset. It would be quite wrong to give the impression that all who suffer from Aids do so as a result of wrongdoing. It is clear that there are sufferers who have contracted the illness through no fault of their own.

Confronted with the complexity of today's crisis, we do well to remember that all is by no means lost. It is still possible for us to draw back from the brink and to lessen, if not entirely eliminate, the menace of the Aids epidemic and indeed to learn from it. In this endeavour we desperately need the knowledge, skills and inventiveness of scientists and doctors. But, more especially, we have to learn how to live and love in a more genuinely human way.

God trusts His people with their moment in history. Our generation has in its hands its own responsibility for the cosmos of which we are part and for the society we are helping to create. In spite of our own mistakes and sins and those of the past, we should never lose hope or faith. We can heal and renew each other if we are prepared to be the embodiment of God's life and love.

It helps to remember that the message of Jesus Christ is that life is to be found in and through death. We are not saved from

1

suffering but through suffering. Disaster, even death itself, carries within itself the promise of resurrection.

This book is of necessity provisional and incomplete. The crisis is new; responses are, as yet, not fully coordinated. That is only to be expected. But a surprising and welcome thing has, I believe, happened. This book, in fact, enlists varied experiences, complementary disciplines, different religions and traditions. From diversity, however, emerges a recognisable unity and a coherent reaction.

I am sure it will meet an urgent pastoral need. It brings together the precious experience of professionals and concerned laity, of religious leaders, priests and religious. It draws on the rich moral heritage of Christian and Jewish traditions. And it makes abundantly clear that the solution to the moral problem which lies behind the questions of public health is not to be found in declarations by experts but in the perceptions and spiritual renewal of the whole people of God. Unless the obvious remedies are vigorously undertaken by the mass of the people, the consequences will be catastrophic and far-reaching.

Gerald Priestland rightly remarks that "When the train has lost its brakes, we have to find ways of stopping it, not just deplore the lack of proper maintenance work in the past". The remedy lies in our hands and the benefit of personal involvement and renewed moral behaviour is to be gained, as Alison Skelton comments, "in personal integrity and in the fine lost art of fidelity".

We cannot yet guess at the magnitude of the crisis which confronts us. Paul Nunn may well be correct in thinking that the known cases represent but "the tip of the iceberg". The response of the Churches will have to be swift, imaginative and radical. Compassion for those who are infected and sick and for their families must go hand in hand with a vigorous and uncompromising campaign to educate those most at risk because of the dangers of sexual irresponsibility.

It is a hard saying but nonetheless true that our future as a society depends on our rediscovery of a strict moral code. We need urgently to live by values which accept that sexual love in its fullness is to be expressed only within life-long and faithful marriage. Only in this way can we safeguard and develop what is noblest and best in human nature.

I pray that this timely book may play a significant part in averting the dangers threatened by the Aids epidemic. It should help professionals and the general public to understand more fully the serious moral issues involved and what needs positively to be done with the utmost energy and determination.

1 Introduction: Why a book on the Church and Aids?

Vicky Cosstick and Timothy Radcliffe OP

Why do we need a book on the Church and Aids? We have heard it said often that there is nothing special about Aids and that, in any event, the problem is a limited one, in the United Kingdom at least. But as we write this introduction over 400 people have died of Aids in the United Kingdom and 735 cases have been diagnosed. Over 5,500 people are known to be carrying the virus and it is possible that by the end of the decade some thousands of people, most of them young, will have died.

Challenge to the Church

From the time of its conception, this book has aimed to be part of the Churches' effort to help people with Aids. It is aimed at any priest or minister, any teacher or adult educator, any doctor or nurse, and any Christian who is concerned directly or indirectly with or about the problem of Aids.

Worries about Aids have been many: what do we as individuals need to know about the disease? In what way will it affect us personally? What are we to think about the disease, and those who have it? How does our Christianity influence what we think? What are we to say about the disease? And what should we do? What *can* we do? Aids has also presented a set of specific questions to the Church. It has challenged our moral theology, our educational systems, our ministry to the sick and the dying, and our expectations of our clergy.

Hardly a day goes by without a mention of Aids in the national papers, and the government has spent millions of pounds on an advertising and information campaign. Yet many of us feel that we still do not know the answers to the questions raised by Aids.

In October 1986, Cardinal Joseph Bernardin, Archbishop of Chicago, wrote in a pastoral letter: "We cannot allow ourselves to identify with only some of the aspects of the Aids phenomenon. We are called to examine more closely *all* its implications." Our response to Aids, he continued, "cannot be fear, ignorance or alienation. . . . We are called, as a community of faith, to confront courageously and compassionately the suffering and death which Aids is bringing to our world."

This book has attempted neither to be fully comprehensive, nor to answer all the questions. In particular, apart from the care-full and stimulating statements by religious leaders, most of the contributions have come from within the Catholic community. But we hope that this book will be seen as one part of the whole Christian response to Aids, while demonstrating some of the particular points of view of Catholics who have thought about Aids, or worked with people with Aids. We also believe that in clarifying the nature of our Christian response we may make a contribution to the wider debate in society.

Through the Christian community

For that reason, the book begins with the basic medical facts about Aids and offers the experience of some individual Aids patients. From that starting point, it moves through the various levels of the Christian community, from the Christian family to the parish, the school, the hospital and the prison, on to consider the areas where the Church meets the secular world. The book ends with pieces by David Alton MP on the government's response and Simon Lee of King's College London on the law.

We have attempted to open up and expand the process of dialogue between and among people with Aids and the Church — by which we mean all the people of God. We have tried to clarify what some of the issues are, to examine them in the light of our faith, and to offer some clues to how Christians might respond. Most of the questions raised may remain unanswered, such as exactly what the Church can do to help those with Aids. That will be up to the individual Christian, in his or her own circumstances. Other questions will remain difficult: just how do we alter the expectations and attitudes of young people towards sexuality?

Cardinal Bernardin, of course, was speaking of the American situation, where over 30,000 cases of Aids have been diagnosed. Some might say that for us in Britain Aids is a limited problem, that relatively few have died in this country and most of those are in London or other major cities. It is not necessarily true that we will be confronted with the tragedy on the same scale.

No delusions

It is possible that Europe has had enough time to avert the worst consequences of the disease—but this does not excuse us from the responsibility of being aware of its global impact. We would also argue that the rest of the country is indeed intimately concerned with the issue of Aids, and with people with Aids. Patients with Aids are going to London—thereby facing automatic joblessness and homelessness in addition to their medical condition—because they believe, erroneously, that medical treatment will be better in the cities, and because they fear isolation within their home communities. They go to London, therefore, not only for medical treatment but to find the support services there.

In reality, the worst thing they can do is to leave home, families and friends. And while most Aids patients are in London, their families come from all over the country. The better informed and more willing to help that the Churches outside the cities are, the more able they will be to offer needed assistance to the medical and other professional agencies. The more willing the Churches are to assist the sick and their families within their own communities, the more likely it is that Aids patients will stay at home, where they can receive the best support and hold on to their jobs and homes.

But let us have no delusions. People with Aids will not walk into their local churches for help. We must shout from the rooftops our willingness to offer whatever support is needed and asked for.

It has frequently been said, and is frequently said in this book, that there is nothing special about Aids. This is as true for the Church as it is for society in general. The Church educates young people, we minister to the sick and dying, we teach a moral viewpoint, we support through our sacraments and community all those who are troubled. While those in secular society often see the Church in terms of its public pronouncements and occasional newsworthy splashes, the clergy and laity are quietly getting on with all these activities in their normal, daily way.

So this book is about all the ordinary, routine activities of the Church in schools, hospitals, parishes and prisons spotlighted, as it were, because of Aids. Aids is special and different because it has presented us with a sudden crisis which demands a response. It calls all these activities into being and challenges them to ensure that they are not just a routine, not just adequate, but that they can meet the challenge.

5

Compassion and the moral tradition

One thing has become clear during the process of putting this book together: the enormous readiness among many people, clergy, religious and laity alike, to help. While the Church may have been accused of being slow off the mark in its response to Aids, the past months have seen conferences and clergy study days held, sex education policies devised, befriending groups formed, special Masses planned.

Nevertheless, Christians can seem rather uncertain about how to respond to Aids. On the one hand there is a clear and indisputable duty to offer compassion to the sick—indeed, "compassion" has become almost a cliché in the context of Aids. Yet the transmission of the virus is usually associated with behaviour that the Church has traditionally condemned: promiscuity, homosexual acts and drug abuse. The Church has aimed, in its public statements, to offer a balance between offering concern and reasserting the Church's traditional teaching, especially since that teaching offers the best protection against infection and the further spread of the virus. And because these two aspects of our response seem to be in tension, the Church can appear not to speak clearly. However well-intentioned, the desire to stand up for our moral tradition appears sometimes to qualify the compassion and make it less than credible.

One way forward is for us to reflect upon what we intend by our statements about morality—and this book aims to help us do that. The Churches are usually associated in the public mind with claims about what is right or wrong. The crisis of Aids invites us to ponder upon how we make moral statements and what we aim to achieve by them. And in this instance we can argue that our desire to be compassionate, to be in solidarity with the sick, cannot be diminished or fudged by our moral views about sexual behaviour, because they both spring from the same root, which is the perception of the goodness of the human body. This is not an abstract theological point, but a recognition of the need to speak clearly and convincingly.

No fundamental tension

All the central and traditional doctrines of Christianity point to the sanctity of the human body. The doctrine of the Incarnation is the belief that God became a human being, took a human body and life as his own; the Eucharist is the celebration of Jesus's offer of his body for our salvation. Belief in the

6

Resurrection springs from the conviction that our bodiliness is so central to who we are that we will only find happiness and fulfillment in God's presence if we are, in some sense, bodily. We are not just minds that could settle for an immortality of the soul. The Church has always clung on to the central belief that our bodies are good and to be cherished. We do not think that it is a good idea to inject heroin or be promiscuous because to live like that would be untrue to our bodiliness, a flight from our humanity.

We believe, and we hope, that this book will demonstrate that there need be no fundamental tension between showing compassion and making moral statements; they ought not to qualify each other since they spring from the same, common and fundamental Christian desire to celebrate our human bodiliness.

In fact, our moral statements will mean little, and may not be heard, unless we are seen to be evidently, obviously, publicly committed to cherishing the bodies of people with Aids. Unless we are seen to be "on the side of" people with Aids, and go out of our way to be in solidarity with them, we might as well not say anything about morality at all. Yet, within the context of caring, our words have a chance of being heard for what they are, as words of healing, words that respect and restore people's dignity.

Called to conversion

One consideration that undoubtedly weighs with Christians is the fear of being misunderstood. If one is seen to be "on the same side" as people with Aids, then one might be thought to approve of all sorts of things, from taking heroin to gay marriage. And one might, understandably, feel that one has a pastoral responsibility to make it known that one does not approve. Yet we run the risk of a different kind of misunderstanding: that it will be thought that our statements about morality are only about approval and disapproval, instead of being about healing and leading human beings to the fullness of life.

In facing the tragedy of Aids, we experience our own vulnerability and powerlessness. And through this, we are called to a "radical conversion", as Fr Bernard Häring says, and offered an opportunity for reconciliation and our own healing. The message that comes through time and time again whenever we listen to those who have worked directly with Aids patients is that in ministering to them we are ourselves ministered to.

At the centre of this book, we hope, you will find the Aids patient himself or herself, with his or her needs, and his or her challenge to the Church. And at the heart of the book, we hope, you will find an invitation. This book, therefore, is about hospitality: it is an attempt to invite all of us to take steps across the threshold into the lives of people with Aids, and to invite them across our threshold. Only when we have clarified the issues for ourselves, when the myths and fears have faded, when we feel confident and fully informed, can we begin to make those steps.

PART I | The medical facts

2 | HIV, Aids and ARC: the virus and the disease

James Bingham

*Director of James Pringle House, the clinic for
sexually transmitted diseases at the Middlesex Hospital*

In mid-1981 cases of a rare pneumonia, due to a protozoan (single cell) organism called Pneumocystis carinii, and a rare skin tumour—Kaposi's sarcoma—were first reported in the United States of America, in California and New York City. Most of the patients were previously healthy homosexual men. These symptoms had been seen before in people who had a deficiency in their immune system, such as patients whose immunity to infections had been deliberately suppressed to prevent organ rejection after kidney transplantation. It was found that the affected group of men were all immune deficient and, by the end of 1981, it was realised that a "new disease"—which became known as the Acquired Immune Deficiency Syndrome (Aids)—had appeared. The first case in Britain was reported in December 1981 at St Thomas's Hospital and cases are being identified in ever-increasing numbers in many parts of the world. The highest prevalence is probably in Central Africa, and from this epicentre it appears to be spreading throughout sub-Saharan Africa.

The causative agent

At first the cause of the condition was unknown, but, as it was very similar to hepatitis B infection epidemiologically, it seemed likely to be due to an infectious agent. A virus was looked for since it was known that certain retroviruses could produce immune suppression in animals. Indeed, a retrovirus, the Human Immunodeficiency Virus (HIV), was identified which is now accepted to be the cause of the condition. Originally, the virus was known as the human T cell lymphotrophic virus type III (HTLV-3) or lymphadenopathy associated virus (LAV).

What does HIV do?

The immune system has two components: the humoral system, which produces antibodies which can attack and neutralise some

11

infections, and the cellular system, where the cells themselves actually deal with the infection. The cells involved are the white blood cells and the particular type are the lymphocytes, the so-called T-lymphocytes. (B-lymphocytes are responsible for producing antibodies.) The virus enters the cells and incorporates its genetic material into that of the lymphocyte. It then replicates within the cell and eventually kills it before moving on to infect further cells. The number of lymphocyte cells are depleted and the cellular immune system becomes deficient, predisposing the sufferer to rare infections and rare tumours.

A new strain of the virus has recently been detected in West Africa and already it has been transmitted, sexually, to Europe. Although a different virus, it produces a syndrome identical to Aids. This virus is known as HIV-2.

The spectrum of HIV infection

It is now realised that HIV infection can produce a wide spectrum of illness. The majority of people are totally unaware of the infection at the time they acquire it. A few experience a glandular fever-like illness, with fever, sweats, enlarged lymph glands and a sore throat, but after this they become, like the others, asymptomatic carriers of the virus and they may remain in this state for some time, perhaps years. Some may go on to develop an intermediate stage of the disease process, the Aids related complex (ARC) and others go on to reach the end stage of the process, Aids. The immune system becomes depleted with the passage of time and a lesser degree of deficiency results in ARC, while a more serious deficiency permits Aids to develop. Many people with ARC will progress to Aids, but a person can present with Aids without apparently having been unwell previously. At first it was believed that about 10 per cent of persons infected with HIV might go on to develop Aids itself; although that figure has now been updated to about 30–35 per cent, with the passage of time it may turn out to be much higher.

The extent of the problem

At first the number of cases of Aids in America doubled every six months, but the doubling time has now slowed to about 11 months. By the end of March 1987, 31,256 cases had been reported in the United States; in Europe the total was 4,000 and

12

in the UK 724 cases had been reported. The extent of the problem is very much greater in parts of Africa, but it is impossible to accurately estimate the number of cases there. While HIV in the industrialised world is a public health emergency, in Africa it has become a public health disaster.

How is the infection spread—and not spread?

The main means of the transmission of HIV infection is by sexual intercourse. The virus can be passed from a man to a woman and from a woman to a man during vaginal intercourse. The main risk activity for homosexual men is anal intercourse and it seems that receptive anal intercourse carries the highest risk. Oral-genital sexual contact is probably not a high risk activity, but as the virus is found in semen and minor damage to the skin may occur, the potential for transmission is there.

From the beginning, HIV infection occurred in haemophiliacs and it was recognised at once that the spread of the virus must be due to something in the blood. In fact, clotting factors such as Factor VIII, which are deficient in haemophiliacs, are obtained from donated blood. It was standard practice to pool the plasma (blood with the red blood cells removed) from many donors, so that a single infected donor could infect a whole pool. By this means, most haemophiliacs in the United States have been infected with HIV. In the UK, about 40 per cent (around 1,000) of haemophiliacs have been infected. The UK now produces its own Factor VIII and no longer obtains it from the United States. It is heat-treated to kill the virus so that further infection by this route should not occur.

If infection can be acquired from blood products it can of course be transmitted from whole blood itself. Before the syndrome was recognised, a small number of people were infected by blood transfusion. All donors now have a blood test for HIV infection performed before their blood is used and this particular problem should now be obviated. The transmission of HIV in the blood also takes place when needles and syringes are shared by intravenous drug abusers.

The final method of transmission is from an infected mother to a child in the womb. It is still not clear whether or not HIV can be transmitted through breast milk; only one case where this might have occurred has been recorded.

Because all donated blood is now tested for evidence of HIV infection anyone requiring a blood transfusion need have no fears about infection. Needles and syringes used for blood tests in hospitals and in general practitioners' surgeries are all disposable and therefore never re-used in this country.

There is no evidence to suggest that the virus is spread by mosquitoes or other insects, in swimming pools, or by sharing cups, eating and cooking utensils, on toilet seats or by sharing air space with an infected person. This is because the virus is extremely fragile and cannot survive for long outside the human body. Much has been said about saliva and the amount of it that may be necessary to transmit the infection. HIV has been isolated in saliva, but infrequently and in very small quantities, and it almost certainly does not represent a risk for transmission. However, most workers in the field would counsel against "French kissing" with an infected person. Infected people should not share razors nor toothbrushes as bleeding may occur during shaving and teeth-cleaning.

There is an overwhelming case against casual contagion and friends and relatives sharing living accommodation are at no risk. Likewise, doctors and nurses, provided they do not come into contact with blood or body secretions, need to take no particular precautions. However, surgeons and laboratory staff who may come into contact with infected blood need to be very careful, especially if they have cuts or abrasions on their hands.

Who gets the disease?

The main group affected in the industrialised world is that of homosexual men. They account for 66 per cent of Aids cases in the United States and 88 per cent of those in the UK. Intravenous drug abusers make up 17 per cent of American cases but only 1.5 per cent of British cases to date, although this is certain to change as large numbers of British addicts are now known to be infected—over 80 per cent of addicts tested in Edinburgh were found to have HIV. Haemophiliacs account for 1 per cent of American cases of Aids, but 4 per cent of British cases; 2 per cent of cases both in the US and in the UK have occurred as a result of transfusion with infected blood, before blood was routinely screened. Four per cent of Aids cases in the United States and 3 per cent of those in the UK have resulted from infection acquired through heterosexual intercourse. If the epidemic spills over into the heterosexual population, the numbers of persons infected with HIV could rise dramatically, as has already occurred in parts of Africa.

In developed countries, haemophiliacs are already known to have infected their partners. It is possible to envisage greater

14

spread into the heterosexual part of the population through intravenous drug abusers, bisexual men and infected prostitutes. It is to be hoped that greater public awareness of the risk may curtail this, but it has already happened. For instance, a young woman, known to me, acquired HIV infection from a bisexual boyfriend with whom she had a sexual liaison as an undergraduate four years ago. He frequently visited New York City and presumably acquired his infection there. The girl has since unfortunately infected her fiancé.

Testing for HIV-infection

In order to prove that someone is infected with HIV it is necessary to take a sample of blood. The laboratory can then examine it for the presence of antibodies to the virus. The test is known as the anti-HIV test. It can easily be performed in one day, unless verification tests have to be performed in equivocal cases. However, it generally takes much longer than a day to obtain the result because of pressure of work on laboratories which have specialised in the test. In the vast majority of people, the test will become positive within three months of infection. Unfortunately, the test does not tell you how long an individual has had the infection, nor does it give any idea as to whether or not the person will go on to develop Aids. It is simply a test that tells you that the person concerned has actually met the virus at some time, but beyond that it is not helpful in establishing a prognosis.

A new test, which measures antigen, is now being developed. It may establish that infection has taken place before an antibody test becomes positive. It is to be hoped that other markers in the blood for the virus will soon be identified and that they might be useful in predicting the course of the infection for the individual. Such markers were discovered for the hepatitis B virus—although it took almost ten years. Not all those who have had hepatitis B are sexually infectious and those that are can now be identified through these serological markers. Most doctors have seen patients with HIV infection or even Aids who have apparently not infected their regular sexual partners, and it is possible that a parallel exists.

How do HIV-infection and Aids present?

As the immune system collapses so the manifestations of HIV infection become apparent. Sufferers may develop minor skin abnormalities, particularly seborrhoeic eczema affecting the face. Thrush in the mouth is common when the patient may complain of a dry mouth, a sore throat or difficulties swallowing. Oral thrush is a clear marker of immune deficiency and therefore a bad sign in terms of prognosis when it develops. Some patients begin to lose weight and this may be associated with diarrhoea for which no obvious cause can be found. Some patients experience night sweats and a flare-up of Herpes simplex (cold sores) and Herpes zoster (shingles). It is usual to monitor the patient's blood as the number of white blood cells may become depleted, as well as the number of platelets, which are essential to prevent haemorrhage. These patients have the Aids related complex (ARC). Many of them are beginning on the slippery slope that terminates with Aids itself.

Patients are diagnosed as having Aids when they develop opportunistic infections or peculiar tumours. Opportunistic infections are rare infections that people with adequate immune systems would not develop. In a short chapter it is not possible to chronicle the full range of infections that exist; the commonest one is a pneumonia caused by an organism called Pneumocystis carinii which may have a slow, insidious onset which is difficult to diagnose. The patient will eventually develop a dry cough and become short of breath, necessitating admission to hospital and, after diagnostic procedures, treatment with intravenous antibiotics. If the diagnosis is made too late the patient may die, but otherwise they usually respond well after a first attack. Patients may also develop a tuberculosis affecting the lung, the bowel or the brain.

Many organisms can affect the bowel but cryptosporidum is the most commonly recognised. It is associated with diarrhoea, which in some cases may be so severe as to cause fluid imbalance, and admission to hospital may be needed to avoid death from dehydration. Treatment is often effective, at least in the short-term.

The nervous system may be affected in patients with Aids. HIV can affect the nerve cells directly and many patients with Aids are now recognised to be suffering from dementia. At present there is no treatment for this. Some peripheral nerves may also be affected. Opportunistic infections of the brain can

16

occur; meningitis due to cryptococcal infection; space occupying lesions due to toxoplasmosis; and tuberculosis and encephalitis due to cytomegalovirus (CMV) infection. CMV can also affect the lungs, the bowel and the retina and may result in blindness unless treated. While many opportunistic infections can be improved with treatment, they are all likely to relapse or the patient may develop more than one infection and perhaps a tumour as well.

Kaposi's sarcoma is the commonest tumour in Aids patients. Patients with KS alone usually have a better prognosis, in terms of longevity, than those with opportunistic infections or both. The lesions are mostly commonly on the skin, are purplish in colour and can spread extensively. They may also be found in the bowel where they may be associated with bleeding. Swelling of the limbs can occur with KS but treatment is most often employed to reduce the size of the lesions on the face where they are highly visible and attract attention. Radiotherapy may be helpful, and in extensive cases chemotherapy and even interferon have been used with some success, although not without unpleasant side effects. Lymphoma, especially affecting the brain, is the other tumour that may be found in Aids patients.

What can be done about Aids?

Although many of the opportunistic infections can be treated and some treatment is available for tumours, at the present time all patients with Aids eventually die. Thus once the end-stage of HIV infection has been reached there is no cure. The course of HIV infection in the early stages probably cannot be influenced either, although a positive psychological approach and healthy living may be of some benefit. It is, therefore, essential that the population as a whole is made aware of the condition and, through a better understanding of the disease, will avoid putting themselves at risk of acquiring the infection.

Through the government's health education campaign, it is to be hoped that most of the comprehending population have got the message; now it is important to ensure that those in the high-risk groups understand the risks. Most homosexual men are well-informed about the problem and have substantially modified their lifestyles. Seroepidemiological studies have shown that in London the percentage of infected homosexual men has not recently increased significantly. This is also true in San Francisco and New York City. Anal intercourse is being avoided by most. Intravenous drug abusers are a more difficult group to reach and the number carrying the virus is increasing.

The prospects for a vaccine

Great efforts are being made to produce a vaccine to prevent further people being infected by HIV. Although some prototypes are presently being tested, it is going to be very difficult to produce a vaccine as the antigenic structure of the virus is constantly changing in a similar way to the influenza virus. Thus the prospects for a vaccine in the near future seem poor.

A number of drugs which directly affect the virus are being tried; the most prominent among them is 5-azido-thymidine (AZT) which is now on the market. The drug works by inhibiting reverse transcriptase, the enzyme necessary for incorporation of the RNA from the virus into the DNA of the lymphocyte. It is being shown that the drug prolongs the life of those who have had Pneumocystis carinii pneumonia and some patients with ARC. It may have considerable side effects including insomnia, muscle aching and profound anaemia. While it is, no doubt, a useful drug, it should be viewed hopefully as the first in a line of anti-viral drugs that may become available. It is unlikely that anti-viral drugs on their own will be the answer and possibly a double approach using an anti-viral and an immune-stimulant may be helpful. Progress is indubitably being made.

3 | Testing, counselling and support

Julia Walters
General practitioner in Northumberland

The Human Immunodeficiency Virus (HIV) has been shown to exist only in the cells and body fluids of human beings. It is fragile and very easily destroyed in those fluids once they leave the host, and no other animal host has been discovered. Tests for antibodies to the virus were introduced around 1984, after the identification of the virus responsible for the medical condition that had become known as Aids. The presence of antibodies in the blood means that the virus has entered the body, has caused the body to react against it, and will persist in the body in the future. Testing has become widely available since then through the National Blood Transfusion Service, sexually transmitted disease clinics, general practitioners, and other specialist hospital departments such as haemophilia clinics.

The "worried-well"

The Department of Health recommendations on testing include a requirement to provide advice and counselling before and after the test, which is allowed only with informed consent. Those who seek the test often do so because they belong to one of the known high-risk groups: homosexuals, intravenous drug abusers and the sexual partners of anyone from these groups or of Africans from the sub-Saharan countries. A large number of people who are in fact at low risk but who think they may be at risk because of their past behaviour may also seek testing. One Aids help-line in the northeast has found that around 50 per cent of its callers belong to this so-called "worried-well" category.

The consultation given before testing needs to take into account the situation of the individual and the degree of his or her risk. The counsellor will also ask about the individual's marital status, the presence of children, employment, social situation, housing, family ties and friendships. Up to three months—or more, in some cases—may elapse between the time of infection and the production of antibodies that can be registered by a positive test result. An individual may be counselled, therefore, to wait before having the test, or to have it repeated later.

The emotions felt by those considering HIV antibody testing will vary, but severe anxiety may occur in total disproportion to the real risk. This anxiety may be so great that it leads to psychiatric symptoms, reactive depression or sleep disorders. It may require treatment with drugs and constant reassurance, even after a negative result. Such symptoms may occur in particular where an individual feels guilty about a sexual liaison outside marriage, often with a prostitute, which is unknown to the spouse. Their anxiety may also produce physical

19

symptoms—such as weight loss, sweating and diarrhoea—which are listed among the non-specific symptoms of Aids itself.

Prolonged follow-up counselling to the test must be available to people, even to those who may have tested negative. Some have great difficulty believing the result and present themselves repeatedly for testing by different agencies. Some have committed suicide because they could not believe the negative result was genuine. Counsellors may ask a clinical psychologist to reinforce their advice and assess whether the client has psychiatric symptoms which require further treatment.

Clearly, people differ in their psychological make-up. Some need to know if they have the virus, while others may have great difficulty coping if the result of the test turns out to be positive. These different attitudes may be reinforced by different counselling agencies. The Terrence Higgins Trust, for example, emphasises the possible disadvantages of testing whereas many sexually transmitted disease clinics are keen to test. Overall, the proportion of tests that turn out positive is very low—about five per cent—and for most people the negative result comes as a great relief. This is very rewarding for the counsellor, who can then offer the client any necessary advice on avoiding the risks in future.

Consequences of a positive result

It is widely accepted at the moment that testing should remain voluntary. Proposals to screen hospital blood samples anonymously to provide further information about the extent of the epidemic are under consideration by the government, but this raises serious ethical and legal dilemmas. Selective testing of other groups, such as ante-natal patients, has also been discussed. If this was done without the informed consent of the patient there would again be major ethical difficulties if antibodies were detected because of the high risk of transmission of the virus to the fetus.

During discussions with the individual, the counsellor will point out other consequences of a positive result. The virus has been found in over 90 per cent of people with a positive antibody test and at present it must be assumed that they are potentially infectious and will remain so for life. They must be advised on how the virus spreads and how to avoid this occurring: they may not donate blood, sperm, body organs or tissue, and should be aware of the transmission of the virus through sexual behaviour and the shared use of intravenous drug abuse equipment.

The risk of developing clinical Aids, for those who are HIV antibody positive, has been estimated at 10–40 per cent. During the medical checks for those who have tested positive, which will usually take place at three-monthly intervals, they will be screened for general symptoms of illness and specific infections, and their immunity levels will be tested. The counsellor will also offer advice to the individual on healthy living, improving diet and exercise, and altering sexual behaviour.

The need for good liaison

Much publicity has been given to the so-called "safer sex" practices, which include use of the condom. Condoms, however, only confer a limited degree of protection and the only totally safe course is sexual abstinence. Many in the high risk groups, such as homosexuals, are already well informed and have shown a high level of responsibility. Others, however, may show a gross disregard for others if they are promiscuous, or are drug addicts financing their habit by prostitution. Even where there is a high level of support in specialised units, drug abusers have a low rate of success in changing their lifestyle.

Counsellors need to have a non-judgmental, genuine, sympathetic and non-possessive attitude towards the people they see. This requires time, flexibility and support from a team of other professionals for the counsellors, who frequently find themselves stressed. Good liaison between the medical teams, community care teams and charities working in the field is also helpful. Confidentiality is absolutely essential in establishing a relationship between the counsellor and the client: because of the widespread anxiety in society about Aids, hostile reactions to the HIV-carrier may still be provoked if news of his or her condition gets out.

In sexually transmitted disease clinics, there is a statutory obligation to maintain confidentiality under the terms of the National Health Service (Venereal Diseases) Regulations (1974), and the staff are experienced at dealing with sensitive and socially unacceptable conditions. Unless the patient specifically requests it, the result of an antibody test will not be released to his or her general practitioner. If the patient develops Aids, however, he or she usually appreciates that the GP should then be informed.

The patient's main fear about informing the GP is usually that it will lead to more widespread disclosures. General practitioners have a duty to ensure that this does not happen,

21

but this can be difficult, partly because secretaries, receptionists and other staff are also members of the local community. Furthermore, insurance companies routinely obtain consent on their proposal forms for medical information to be released, and their forms may now include a specific question about Aids and Aids related conditions. Some insurance companies require all single men to have a blood test or ask the GP if they think the patient is a homosexual. No insurance company will accept anyone who is antibody positive for life insurance, and so no mortgage will be possible.

Turning for support to the family

During the first flush of emotion on hearing that the test result is positive, an individual will need a great deal of support. Their first reaction may be denial or blank disbelief; they may be devastated and tearful. They may be predominantly fearful of the effect of the test result on their relationships. Or they may from the beginning be quite philosophical. They will often turn for support first to their families, especially where family ties are strong, and particularly outside London. Telling others, however, is risky, and caution is advised. There is no need to tell an employer and most people try to avoid this for fear of the panic that may occur among colleagues and clients.

For these reasons, it is important that any follow-up counselling and medical checks should be done conveniently, with a minimum of waiting for appointments, and that it does not entail time off from work. With the increasing number of patients at some clinics, this is becoming a problem. Dentists should be told so that they can take a few basic precautions— but there have been occasions where dentists refused to treat HIV-carriers or have taken extreme measures, such as displaying large warning notices in waiting areas and wearing crash helmets to protect their eyes!

Haemophiliacs were among the first to be screened for HIV antibodies. They often came from families where more than one member was infected. When they discovered that many of them were infected by the contaminated Factor VIII they felt great anger and this affected the long-term relationships of trust that had previously existed between them and the staff at the haemophilia clinics. They needed opportunities to express their anger and fear, as individuals and in groups, and have been helped by the openness of staff and being informed of the medical facts as they have emerged.

22

Support for those with faith

Charities such as the Terrence Higgins Trust and Aids North have set up self-support groups for those who are HIV-carriers which can offer great help. Some gain from the feeling that they can help others after they have adjusted to the news of their own condition. Both these organisations have subgroups catering to those with religious affiliations. The Interfaith Group in London, for example, maintains a confidential, nationwide list of clergy who are available for spiritual counselling or the sympathetic taking of funerals. Members of these church groups also help by educating other Christians, supporting those engaged directly in pastoral work, with people with Aids, and requesting prayers from church leaders.

When a patient who is HIV-positive develops Aids or ARC they are, at present, likely to be treated in an ordinary hospital. Because they have often experienced rejection, patients need a very positive approach from medical staff. The care of Aids patients requires a consciously open, friendly and sympathetic attitude, especially on first meeting. Initially this may be difficult for staff, who must overcome thir own fears, prejudices and even ignorance. If an initially positive attitude is reinforced by listening, caring and non-judgmental discussion, then a relationship of trust will develop.

Aids is a fatal condition, and though its course varies, most, once diagnosed with "full-blown" Aids, have died within two years. The situation for people with Aids is very different from that of those suffering from other terminal conditions such as cancer. Cancer patients usually receive strong support from their families and friends, and they in turn support each other. Society's attitude to cancer is sympathetic and charities receive a great deal of money. Although Aids patients do often turn to their immediate families for support and often return from London or abroad to spend the last phase of their illness with them, the extended family is usually not informed or involved. Secrecy is maintained not only because of the fear of an immediate negative response but because the patient fears that prejudice will continue after his or her death towards the surviving members of the immediate family.

Stress for the medical staff

The lack of opportunity for the close family and especially the parents of Aids patients to discuss their child's illness places

23

great stress on them. After admission to hospital the nursing staff must spend a great deal of time listening to and supporting the family as well as the patient. Nurses can become very involved emotionally with the patients and their families, leading to stress among the medical staff. Patients who have not shared the diagnosis with their families may have only the nursing and other medical staff, and sometimes their gay partners, to support them.

There is a considerable geographic variation in the problems that patients face. Homosexuals and drug addicts in some major cities may have the added problems of poor housing, material poverty, under-nourishment and general ill-health, in addition to the lack of family support. Any form of community care must take these factors into account and involve a wide group of people to continue the treatment initiated in hospital and provide social and financial support. Aids patients may have difficulty in claiming the range of state benefits—attendance and mobility allowances, special help with the cost of heating and diet—to which they are entitled because of their condition. Each allowance must be claimed separately and the diagnosis must be disclosed on each occasion.

Before community care can successfully be achieved, there is much mythology about Aids which will need to be dispelled by better education. Sadly, even those who have access to the correct information frequently do not bother to absorb it or continue to act in ignorance of the facts. The Royal College of Nursing has produced guidelines for the care of Aids patients but some nurses remain ignorant of them and try to avoid contact with people with Aids.

Doctors, surgeons, dentists and laboratory staff have also received guidance on how to deal with patients with HIV infection which emphasise a high standard of clinical practice to avoid the risk of infection. If such standards are maintained there will be no need for a "plague mentality" or leper-like isolation since there will be no need to distinguish between people with Aids and other patients.

The scope of the Aids problem is likely to increase in the next few years and it is likely that most people will eventually come into direct contact with the problems themselves. The experience of those who have already been involved may help every individual to respond in a responsible and humane way.

4 | Aids and the developing world

Paul Nunn
Lecturer at the London School of Hygiene and Tropical Medicine

Aids is now recognised to be a major global health problem and the World Health Organisation (WHO) and its member states are mobilising resources throughout the world to combat its spread. Yet of the 45,608 cases reported by 102 countries to WHO by the end of March 1987, 73 per cent were from the United States alone, over 10 per cent from Europe and only some 15 per cent from the whole of the developing world. At first sight these figures would suggest that Aids is a problem predominantly of the West and not one that need bother those concerned about the health of people in Africa, South America or Asia. In this chapter I shall argue the reverse, namely that Aids is already a considerable problem for some of these countries and likely to have far-reaching consequences for their development.

I must first point out, however, that hard data relating to the impact of Aids on the developing world is very sparse. What little does exist is largely derived from selected groups and of limited applicability to the population as a whole. There is a great need to obtain accurate information not only on the spread of HIV in developing countries but on mortality and morbidity from all causes. It is impossible to predict what effect Aids will have on the young adult population, for example, if we do not yet know the factors already affecting it. I will therefore first lay out the facts concerning the spread of Aids in the developing world and especially Africa and then attempt, more by crystal-ball gazing than by analysis of existing data, to assess the impact this will have on these countries.

Aids in Africa

The African connection with Aids was first established in Belgium in the early 1980s when it became apparent that Africans were seeking treatment for a condition with many

25

similarities to that described in young homosexual men in the United States and which subsequently became known as Aids. This prompted American and Belgian investigators to look for the disease in Africa itself in patients who had never been elsewhere. Their findings, published in 1983, clearly showed that the disease was established there as in the West. Subsequent work outlined the differences and the similarities between African and US/European Aids.

First, HIV is the cause of Aids in Africa as it is in the West. Although African strains have slight structural differences compared to Western isolates these do not significantly alter their behaviour. New viruses related to but distinct from HIV have been reported from West Africa. At least one of these (HIV-2) causes a disease currently indistinguishable from Aids.

Second, epidemiological research showed that the Aids epidemic in Africa differs from that in Europe and the United States by being predominantly caused by heterosexual intercourse. Our current level of knowledge suggests that homosexuality is extremely rare in Africa apart from a few instances where it is an accepted part of the culture in small and relatively isolated communities such as the Swahili in Mombasa. Intravenous drug abuse, the second commonest risk factor in the West, is virtually unknown in sub-Saharan Africa outside the Republic of South Africa. However, materno-fetal transmission and blood transfusion are major routes of infection because many more women of child-bearing age are infected, and in most African countries screening of donated blood occurs only in the major centres if at all. The exact percentage of cases of Aids and of HIV carriers infected by these means in Africa is not known but will probably vary from place to place.

There are haemophiliacs in Africa, but they are less common than in the West. Patients with sickle-cell disease are an equivalent group, however, since they frequently receive blood transfusions and Aids has indeed been reported among them. Poorly sterilised needles and syringes may play a part in the transmission of HIV, but this needs to be confirmed. It is even less certain what role ritual scarring of the body and circumcision, both male and female, might play in the transmission of HIV, but they are potential risks.

The profound impact of Western research

It can be seen then that apart from children receiving blood transfusions, the majority of the at-risk population are either infants or sexually active adults. Almost all cases of Aids in Africa fall into these two groups. This is the strongest evidence we have against insect transmission, the method apparently of most concern to Westerners. Neither has work on insects shown that transmission from insects to people is even possible under normal circumstances.

Third, it is important also to mention work by Western researchers which gave false results and is already having profound adverse effects on the further understanding and limitation of the spread of HIV in Africa. The first was a study of serum taken during the 1960s from children in the West Nile district of Uganda which purported to show evidence of HIV in many of the samples tested. This implied that HIV had been present for some time in this population and that some individuals were immune to it. It also gave rise to the idea that this population, or one like it elsewhere in Africa, may have been the origin of the Aids epidemic. Unfortunately the test used in this work gave high numbers of false positive results. In other words, the samples appeared to be infected with HIV when they were not. The same test was used in a number of surveys throughout Africa. By the time it became obvious that these mistakes had been made, Africa had already been labelled in the public mind in the West as the source of Aids. Understandably, many African states reacted by refusing to admit the existence of an "Aids problem", withdrawing cooperation from expatriate research groups, and delaying the implementation of prevention programmes.

Estimating the number of HIV-infected

So what is the true scale of the Aids epidemic in Africa? As we know, the number of actual cases of Aids gives only a very incomplete picture of the whole epidemic; they are only the "tip of the iceberg". In developing countries the lack of resources to diagnose either HIV-infection itself or the opportunistic infections that it causes, quite apart from any political reluctance to report cases, make the reported figures even more of an underestimate. Nevertheless, some 3,500 cases of Aids had been reported to WHO by African states up to the end of March 1987.

Of much greater relevance to an estimate of the size of the problem is the number of people infected with HIV. Surveys conducted using reliable tests give results varying from 1 per cent of 1200 people in the Cameroons to 18 per cent of blood

27

donors in Kigali, Rwanda. However, blood donors are far less representative of the general public in Africa than in Europe. If it is true that HIV infection is more common among the educated classes and in the urban areas as has been claimed, then figures derived from blood donors may give a misleadingly high figure since donors tend to be in employment, in towns, and better educated. Among more than 2,000 employees in a Kinshasa hospital 6 to 7 per cent were found to be infected with HIV. In comparison, the rate of infection among military recruits to the United States armed forces was about 0.15 per cent of over 300,000 tested. Studies among people attending sexually-transmitted disease clinics and prostitutes show an even higher rate of infection, and recent work in Kenya shows the speed with which the virus can spread through a population. Four per cent of female prostitutes tested in Nairobi were positive for HIV in 1980–81, 51 per cent in 1983–84, and 59 per cent in 1985–86. This shows how vulnerable prostitutes are to infection and also how instrumental they may be in passing it on. Among hospital employees in Kinshasa the rate of acquisition of infection was much lower (0.8 per cent per annum).

WHO's admittedly very crude estimate of the total number of people infected in Africa is two million, but the true figure could exceed five times this.

Aids in the remainder of the developing world

Information from other parts of the developing world is much harder to come by. Brazil ranks third in the list of countries reporting Aids cases, behind the United States and France, and there the epidemic seems to be following the US/European pattern, with homosexuality and drug abuse being the main risk factors. Haiti leads the Caribbean states with 785 cases reported by the end of 1986. Relatively small numbers of cases have been reported from the other South American states, the Indian subcontinent, South East Asian states and Oceania.

Although some surveys among high-risk groups such as prostitutes have been published in the medical press, it seems likely that other developing countries have learnt the disadvantages of publicity relating to Aids from the experience of some African states, and are keeping quiet. Very often where cases of Aids are reported it is with the "disclaimer" that they are members of some immigrant group who have brought the disease in from elsewhere.

The impact of Aids

Dealing first with the individual, the diagnosis of Aids or of HIV infection is clearly a shattering blow which will be dealt with differently by different personalities. In Africa, however, myths and rumours circulate which may influence the individual's response and rebound again on society. For example, it is reported that in Zambia a widely held myth is that the cure for Aids is to have sex with a virgin.

The practical implications of Aids in a young adult are often different from those in the West. Anyone with a steady job in Africa is likely to be supporting not only his or her own spouse and children, but many other dependents as well. More people than the immediate nuclear family, therefore, are likely to suffer from the loss of a wage-earner.

The institution of the extended family is also threatened by Aids: grandparents may be left with large numbers of dependent children to care for following the loss of the intervening generation. The rapidity with which this may happen, the attendant grief and the economic burden may mean that the grandparents are unable or unwilling to take on this responsibility. Even if they do, the economic resources available for a given child are likely to be considerably less. Whole families will become much poorer. If the surviving relatives do not shoulder the burden then the responsibility for the care of children will be shifted to the wider community or even the state. Thought needs to be given to the provision of orphanages or other locally acceptable forms of care.

In the rural areas, young adults supply not only the family income but also the labour for producing food. The effects of their loss if the seed cannot be sown or the produce harvested are likely to be more immediate than in the towns. Malnutrition, its related diseases and even starvation may therefore increase. A loss of agricultural production will in turn affect urban society, food prices will rise, malnutrition will also increase in the towns, and there will be pressure especially on the young men who have gone there for study or work to return to the country to farm vacant land.

In increasingly Westernised African society, young adults hold crucial economic and administrative positions. Material development will be jeopardised not only directly by the deaths of employees, but also by the commitments to life and health insurance offered by employers in industry and government who did not foresee the significant mortality. It is much more

29

imperative to attend the funerals of friends and even distant relatives in Africa than in the West and the rituals go on for longer. Some firms in Zaire, for example, are having to limit the amount of time employees can spend attending these obsequies.

The impact on health care

Roughly one quarter to one third of babies born to HIV-infected mothers will also be infected and likely to die within two years of birth. The impact this will have on birth rates and population will depend above all on what percentage of mothers becomes infected. It may also be influenced by the reaction of young people and women especially to the increase in child mortality: some, particularly HIV-infected women, may avoid pregnancy (there is some reason to believe that progress of the disease may worsen during pregnancy); others may react by having more children. There is clearly a risk that advances in child health and the rates of survival of infants gained over the past 20 years will be negated by Aids.

Further advances in general health from expanded immunisation programmes, the extension of primary health care and so on that might reasonably have been anticipated in developing countries in the next few years will also be undermined by the redirection of resources from current programmes to those dealing with Aids.

In the absence of an effective vaccine or treatment for Aids, education and the screening of donated blood become the only means of limiting the spread of HIV infection. Health education, previously a neglected, under-valued and under-resourced part of health care, will receive more resources. If correctly handled this may have some advantages: the Western concept of health care, which depends on drugs, hospitals and expensive facilities, may be seen to be less infallible and more emphasis may be placed on the community or the individual's own responsibility for creating and maintaining his or her health.

Attempts will undoubtedly be made by some states to prevent the entry of HIV carriers. This has already happened in countries such as India, where a policy of screening all African students has been adopted. At present this contravenes international regulations governing the freedom of movement of individuals and, in any case, is likely to be a useless exercise in all but those states that have a very low incidence of HIV infection. However, it is clearly not in the interests of a developing country to spend scarce resources on a student with

30

a limited life expectancy. Countries may therefore themselves voluntarily screen students before sending them abroad for further studies.

Implications for the developed world

One immediate possibility is that Aids could become established in the heterosexual population in the West just as it has in Africa. However, we do not know the necessary conditions for such a shift in the pattern of the disease and only further research in those areas where heterosexual transmission is the norm will reveal these. It is therefore imperative that the rifts between the West and African and other developing countries, caused by inaccurate early research work and the perception on both sides that Africa is somehow "to blame" for Aids, be repaired.

On a wider front it should be accepted that Aids is a global problem and that global solutions offer the only chance of success in preventing its spread. Judgmental and critical attitudes towards the way developing countries are handling their Aids problems should be replaced by offers of aid in the form of experienced personnel, equipment and materials to detect HIV infection and assess the scale of the epidemic in the country concerned, and to provide care for those suffering from the disease. Pressure on governments will be required to encourage such aid and other fund-raising bodies need to raise public awareness. The Churches should overcome their scrupulous reluctance to become involved in Aids. International collaboration between agencies is as essential as between donor nations and recipients and many look to WHO to form the network of collaboration that will be required to defeat the worst pandemic that most people on earth today have ever faced.

5 | Mothers and babies

John Osborne
Consultant gynaecologist at the Middlesex Hospital

Before we consider the ways in which Aids may affect the mother and child, before and after birth, we must realise that we are not just considering women who have been diagnosed as having Aids, but also any woman carrying the HIV virus. Women with clinically diagnosed Aids will already be under the care and treatment of a specialist.

HIV infection is not the only viral illness that a mother may contract which is capable of affecting the unborn child; for example, rubella (German measles) still causes congenital abnormalities. Nor is it the only sexually transmitted disease that may be passed on to a child—syphilis caused many unborn children to be infected before the discovery of adequate treatment with antibiotics.

The special problems with regard to HIV-infection concern not only the possibility that the virus may be transmitted to the child. If the child is infected, the virus may remain with the child throughout its life, he or she may die of the disease, or, if not, pass it on to the next generation. In addition, the HIV-infected mother is at risk because her condition may deteriorate as a result of being pregnant.

At the outset it must be admitted that because this is a relatively new problem accurate figures with regard to numbers of cases and risks are woefully inadequate. As yet there do not appear to be many female carriers of the virus (other than in certain high risk groups) in the Western world and figures from Africa must be interpreted in the light of the lack of resources available there to investigate the problem.

How many women are carriers?

Because full population screening has not been undertaken we can only by indirect means obtain an idea of the number of women infected. In the United States, 0.1 per cent of blood donors are infected but, because those in high risk groups are discouraged from donating blood, this is probably an underestimate. Figures for the prevalence of HIV in high risk groups are very variable: studies in the United States have indicated that between 2 and 59 per cent of intravenous drug abusers are infected and between 3 and 40 per cent of female prostitutes. In the United Kingdom, the number of reported cases of HIV infection in women has risen rapidly, with a 26 per cent rise since 1 January, 1987. At the end of February the total number was 210, but this is probably also an underestimate.

What is the magnitude of risk to the mother?

To consider the risk to the mother or the potential mother one must first understand that HIV affects her immune system, which fights infection and resists malignant changes. Pregnancy also affects the immune system, adapting the mother to allow a "foreign being", the baby, to develop within her body. This combination of HIV infection and pregnancy would appear, in some cases, to combine such that the risk of a woman infected with HIV progressing to the disease of Aids seems to be increased by her becoming pregnant. In short, pregnancy may cause a woman to progress more quickly to Aids, which is, at present, in the end universally fatal.

In a small American study 33 per cent of HIV-positive women developed Aids within 30 months of delivery; a further 47 per cent developed Aids related conditions; and only 20 per cent were symptom free. This suggests a significantly increased risk to the mother above the risk if she had not had a baby.

Risk to the child

In considering the risks to the baby, one must try and assess what the chances are of the baby receiving the virus from its mother. Studies, particularly in Africa, suggest that 50 per cent of babies born to women who are HIV-positive will also have positive tests. They may not all harbour the virus but certainly some may die of Aids in the neonatal period. We do not yet know what will happen to those who have the virus as they grow up but the virus's effect on brain tissue could be serious. There have also been reports that the virus may affect the development of the baby in the womb, leading to abnormalities and a failure to grow at the expected rate.

Figures for children under 13 with HIV infection in the United States show that 76 per cent of them had, as their only risk factor, mothers in a high risk group while 18 per cent appear to

33

have been infected by blood transfusion. Forty-eight per cent of the mothers were intravenous drug abusers and 10 per cent of the mothers had sexual partners who were bisexual or intravenous drug abusers.

In the United Kingdom the figures for children under 15 are different. Of 117 reported cases, 104 are haemophiliacs, one is a recipient of blood products, 10 were born to HIV-positive mothers and two are from Africa. This apparent preponderance of blood products as a source of infection will probably change with the screening of blood and its products and the rise in the number of HIV-positive women.

The high risk mothers are: women with evidence of Aids or ARC; intravenous drug abusers; women from countries where heterosexual transmission of HIV infection is common (mainly central Africa); and the female sexual partners of intravenous drug abusers, bisexual men, haemophiliac men, men with Aids and men from countries where heterosexual transmission of the virus is common.

Because of the known risk, the testing of all pregnant women has been suggested, but this raises practical, moral and ethical questions. Certainly a screening programme would provide us with accurate figures about the numbers of infected people, but what should we do about mothers-to-be with positive tests? There is at present no effective treatment to offer pregnant women with HIV infection and we can only tell them the quite serious potential problems for them and their child.

What counselling can be offered? It may seem extreme but one has to say that the best advice that can be given to a woman who is infected with HIV is that with the present lack of treatment it would be best for her if she never becomes pregnant. This may be drastic but one has to consider that there is a very high risk that the baby may be infected. If the mother progresses to develop Aids herself this unfortunate child may also be left motherless, with the added stigma of carrying the virus. Women who are infected with HIV should also be warned not to donate blood or tissue, and encouraged to persuade their sexual partners to be tested.

Practical advice for mothers

The woman who is HIV infected and pregnant needs good antenatal care in the same way as any other mother, with an emphasis on assessing the child's development in the womb. The added precautions necessary for the attendant at the birth may mean the isolation of the mother in labour, but except for blood contact at that time the virus is not highly contagious.

After birth the baby must be tested but it will be some time before it is definitely known whether or not the baby has acquired the virus. It is probably wiser for the baby to be bottle rather than breast fed as there have been case reports of babies acquiring the virus, which may appear in breast milk, after birth. Otherwise the mother and baby should be encouraged to behave as normally as possible to encourage bonding under what must be difficult circumstances.

After the mother has given birth the discussion must inevitably turn to the future, and the decision on whether she should risk another pregnancy. This will require careful and sympathetic counselling involving the family unit, the medical team caring for her, and religious advisers, because the future of all those in the family may be affected.

One new virus, HIV-2, has already been identified and others may well follow. Continuous vigilance by virologists will be required to keep ahead of the changes and develop new tests. Every new disease presents us with challenges but few have the potential for damage to future generations. The spread of HIV in women has begun in the United Kingdom and appears to be rapidly increasing. We must monitor the spread to enable us to assess when general screening of pregnant women may be required. The challenge to society is to protect the next generation. This will require changes in the sexual attitudes and practices that have been widely accepted over the past two decades.

PART II | People with Aids

6

The path to reconciliation

David Forrester
Portsmouth Roman Catholic diocesan Aids director

Robert—a pseudonym—is a university graduate, aged 23, who lives a long way from home. He is handsome, highly intelligent, sensitive and gifted. When he obtained his degree, his teachers predicted a brilliant future for him. Four months ago Robert was screened at a clinic for sexually transmitted diseases and diagnosed HIV-positive. This means that he will be a carrier of the virus for the rest of his life, and may at some unknown stage go on to develop full-blown Aids.

The authors of *Aids: The story of a disease*, John Green and David Miller, describe the test Robert took as "something of a Pandora's box". There is no treatment and no way of knowing whether Robert will go on to develop Aids. In the Greek myth, at least hope remained in Pandora's box after it had been rashly opened and all human ills had been dispersed to play havoc among mankind. For Robert, however, the test result was devastating; it seemed to remove even hope.

Precisely because Robert is unusually gifted, he knew more than most the implications of the test result. He had heard how people like himself had suffered discrimination at work, been denied life insurance, found it difficult to obtain a mortgage, and had been the butt of abuse and a fair measure of prejudice and hysteria. In a sense, he was prepared and knew he would have to cope with the stigma attached to being a carrier of the virus. What he had not reckoned with was his own reaction to the news. In retrospect, there are times when Robert even now wonders whether it would have been wiser not to take the test.

The news that he was HIV-positive was particularly painful for Robert because, despite all his talents, for most of his life he has had a poor self-image. He constantly under-valued his true worth. He was brought up by an exceedingly loving mother, but a distant father, and this imbalance in the manner in which as a child he had received love and his sense of worth and security appears to have strengthened an early disposition towards homosexuality. When he was a teenager, his parents divorced and, almost inevitably, he took the side of his mother, which caused further emotional scars, especially those of guilt. From there it was a short step to self-hatred. As Robert told me:

> When I was 13 I started praying that God would make right my sexuality. This I continued until I was 18. I prayed every night, pleading with him because I thought God could do anything. I stupidly made bargains with him. I told him I couldn't cope and I needed his help. In my heart I knew I was not a bad person. I didn't say "To hell with it" and turn my back, until the end, in desperation.

This last phrase referred to the occasion at university when Robert had finally allowed himself to be seduced by an older man. Instead of bringing Robert the least satisfaction, this experience only increased—as he knew it would—his self-contempt. Robert then attempted suicide. Ironically, Robert did not die, but instead, and from that one and only affair, became infected with the HIV virus. To guilt Robert now added despair:

> At first I thought that Aids would make little difference. I had never been happy, so one more burden should be easy to accept and besides, it was a wish come true (or an answered prayer). But now I think it is all too much. My world and its possibilities are shrinking at a time when they should have been expanding. It's OK for T. S. Eliot to "rejoice that things are as they are" (*Ash Wednesday*). At least he had known "the power of the usual reign", the glory of the "positive hour".
> . . . I'm not at all sure I've had that pleasure.

It is now four months since Robert was diagnosed HIV-positive and I came to know him. These days he prays a great deal, frequently attends Mass, and has requested me to give him instruction in the Faith. Nevertheless, it should not be assumed that the Church has no more to do except receive him, like any other convert, into her midst. What about his poor self-image and the anger which frequently engulfs him? What is the Christian response to an outburst such as this?

> I am consumed with anger; angry with the world, God and myself. I am livid, while you try and talk reason . . . as if things are not as bad as they seem. That among other things makes me want to unleash my fury on you. On you and God . . . you all serve to remind me that I am a dreadful person. I am numb to love. I just feel pain, a deep, resentful pain.

A seamless robe

In the light of how Robert occasionally regards himself, it is important that any Christian seeking to relate to him and others like him should remember that the extent to which we accept and forgive ourselves is the real extent to which we can genuinely accept and forgive our neighbour. Indeed it is also the extent to which we understand the love, acceptance and forgiveness of God. Love, acceptance and forgiveness are a seamless robe.

It is simply not Christian to exclude oneself from God's compassion whilst proclaiming it is bestowed on all others. Similarly there is no virtue in harbouring hatred and contempt for oneself while attempting to love one's neighbour. To do so is to deny that we are all made in the image of God. These truths, lived out in practice, are paramount when relating to anyone either infected with HIV or an actual sufferer of Aids or ARC.

Robert's situation also illustrates vividly the fallacy of assuming that all those infected with HIV or who have Aids have necessarily led promiscuous lives. Robert has had only one sexual relationship in his whole life, and that occurred only after years of self-torture, when he was literally at his wit's end. What makes his particular suffering all the sadder, however, is the fact that, unlike so many of his peers, Robert remained chaste for so long because of his firm belief that sexual intercourse should be an expression of love and not entered into simply to fulfil one's sexual appetites. Had things been different, there is nothing he would have liked better than to have married, striven to have loved his wife faithfully, and to have had children. More than a few of his contemporaries find his view of sex either old-fashioned or too idealistic. In reality it is Christian.

Even now Robert remains convinced of this, which is partly why he feels so ashamed and is anxious for God's forgiveness. It is here that the Church is able to reassure him and remind him of Christ's testimony that whoever sins the most and is pardoned goes on to love the most (Lk 7.36-50). The healing ministry of the Church in situations like this cannot be exaggerated. It is especially the duty of the Church to dispel the notion that Aids has anything to do with divine retribution. As Robert said:

It is difficult enough to come to terms with the guilt and anger which I feel, knowing the disease is in a sense self-inflicted, without being burdened with the idea that as a homosexual I have been singled out by God to receive punishment as a sinner. Sufferers need to be reassured that this is not the view held by the Church, but only that of the misinformed.

41

Breaking the news

Robert has discovered, however, that among Christians forgiveness is usually something that follows acceptance. This was certainly the rewarding lesson that he learned when he travelled home to break the news of his condition to his mother and father, and seek a reconciliation with the latter. Robert found both his parents in their different ways remarkably understanding, albeit upset. There were no reactions of disgust, recrimination, fear or rejection. This at least partly convinced him that he was in fact loved and lovable, and perhaps not the totally dreadful person he had imagined himself to be for so long.

His closest friend reacted in precisely the same way. If anything it deepened the friendship, which had already weathered Robert's announcement that he was homosexual and had had an affair with an older man. To this, Robert's friend had instinctively reacted as a practising Catholic should. To what extent this influenced Robert to seek instruction in the Catholic faith we shall probably never know. Certainly it was because of the compassionate but unsentimental approach of his Catholic friend that Robert was prepared to meet and talk with me.

It seemed vital to establish right from the start what Robert expected from a Catholic counsellor. For that reason, while travelling to London with Robert for a meeting called to discuss the recruitment, selection and training of counsellors for Aids sufferers and carriers of the virus, I deliberately asked him what qualities he would look for in a counsellor—as distinct from someone who might wish to befriend a sufferer and lend a hand with practical matters.

A good listener

Robert was exceedingly quick to say that "a counsellor must *not* be someone jolly!" Such a person should be a good listener, he thought. He was most anxious that the counsellor should be able to empathise, in other words be able to place himself or herself in the shoes of the person they were seeking to counsel. Robert also wanted a counsellor to be prepared to express his or her feelings, especially those of compassion, including to the point of weeping when so inclined. Obviously he expected a counsellor not to be prejudiced or judgmental. He was particularly anxious that a Catholic counsellor should proclaim that genuine Christian compassion surpassed all moral judgments. For that same reason, and to avoid hindering the growth of the sufferer's relationship with either God or the counsellor, Robert was anxious that the latter should not be concerned with the extraction of "confessions". He also wished a counsellor to possess self-knowledge and an integrated personality, as well as knowledge of the disease.

What Robert failed to mention was the need for the counsellor to be tough, to be able to keep one's balance and not cave in under the constant demands of trying to bring hope to people under threat of death. With a little prompting, however, he did concede that counselling a person such as himself might be quite exhausting, given his particular tendency to oscillate between extreme depression and pessimism and relatively positive thinking. Robert began to appreciate that working with dying young people might be a desperate experience and, in important ways, different from dealing with those who suffer from terminal illnesses to which there is no stigma attached as in Aids. He saw how it could be capable of producing in such workers tremendous feelings of anger, sadness and helplessness, the danger of "burnout", and the need for counsellors to have the support of their colleagues.

Purpose and meaning in staying alive

It was probably from that point that Robert began to experience a slow, often painful but steady change in his outlook. Despite occasional regressions, he began to become more positive. Instead of always giving in to understandable feelings of despair, he discovered that he could be of value to others. Incidentally, what Robert may never appreciate is the joy I felt from the time when I first perceived tentative signs of self-worth developing in him, as well as the growth of a positive will to stay alive as long as possible—in order to be of service to others.

Like countless other people suffering from a possibly terminal condition, Robert is now gradually finding a purpose and meaning for staying alive by attempting to alleviate the heartache and pain of those men and women in situations worse than his own. His growing Christian conviction that life here on earth is but a foretaste of eternal life, where there is no more suffering, tears or sadness, is contributing enormously to this positive change in his outlook. He is naturally still fearful of the process of death, but death itself no longer frightens him. In this Robert has been assisted by his view of the faith and how he regards the Church:

43

On discovering that I was HIV-positive, the realisation suddenly dawned on me that I am mortal. I might not have the time to fulfil my plans and ambitions and those many things which I have put off until tomorrow. I have had to search more vigorously for the meaning of life—if life has no meaning then there is no point to suffering and surviving. For me the answer is provided in Christianity.

In God the Father I find a sense in suffering. In Jesus Christ I find the inspiration to accept the challenge of suffering. In the Holy Spirit I find the strength and courage to face and fight suffering. The Church is a structure to support me in this fight, providing compassion and encouragement and perhaps practical help if I were to fall ill.

In the field of practical help Robert was quite clear that the Church had a specific role to play:

I would look to the Church to supplement the care and healing offered by the health service. This healing would obviously centre on the spiritual and mental well-being of the sufferer, but also, in the absence of a medical cure, some thought could be given to releasing his spiritual potential by faith in Jesus Christ to fight the effects of the virus. The sacraments of Anointing the Sick and the Holy Eucharist can fortify and sustain the sufferer and can be regarded as additional weapons in his fight against Aids. If the disease progresses to the terminal stages, then a Church-organised hospice would perhaps be particularly comforting as a patient prepares to die.

Without doubt, when sufferers from Aids and carriers of the virus such as Robert seek help from the Church, most of them are essentially seeking a meaning to life and either the will to struggle on or the courage to face death. In that we are all brothers and sisters. As Victor Frankl once remarked:

For too long we have been dreaming a dream from which we are now awakening: the dream that if we just improve the socio-economic situation of people, everything will be okay, people will become happy. The truth is that as the *struggle for survival* has subsided, the question has emerged: *survival for what*? Ever more people today have the means to live, but no meaning to live for.

(V. Frankl, *The Unheard Cry for Meaning*, 1979)

With the onset of Aids it is even more imperative that the Church should provide the world, and not least people such as Robert, with the meaning of life found in the Gospel.

7 | Speaking personally: four people with Aids

edited by Vicky Cosstick

Andrew, aged 32

I first learned I was antibody positive when I took a test in July 1985 at a clinic I attended regularly. The counselling service at Westminster Hospital was very good. They explained very clearly what being antibody positive meant. It didn't surprise me in one respect. My lifestyle might have led me to believe that I was a candidate for Aids.

There was only one thing I could do. I couldn't tell anyone that I was HIV-positive (some people find it easy, but I just couldn't), and so I just stopped having sex. It was difficult at first, but I have found that I could live without it. I didn't grow two heads or anything, I'm still smiling, and I've gone on enjoying everything I enjoyed before. The thought I couldn't bear, and I try not to think about it now, is that I might have infected someone else before I took the test . . .

I felt fine that year. I started a new job managing a theatre. It was a job I very much wanted and I really committed myself to it, but it was very stressful, up to 100 hours a week, and I laid myself wide open to the disease. I developed pneumonia in June 1986 and was told after a week in hospital that I had Aids.

Things were very bad and I got very down. What kept me going was the communion brought to me every day in hospital by Alex, a friend of mine who's a priest. This was an immense support to me. Its effect was literally physical, and made me able to cope. The worst thing then was telling my mother—it just broke her heart—and my friends. But I haven't had a bad reaction from anyone, just shock because it's such an extremely unpleasant disease. I think the gutter press have been criminally irresponsible over Aids, which is a disease that is not contagious. Aids is not like TB or hepatitis. What we need is peace, the love of friends and family, and a job if we're capable of doing it. The very thing we need we have been denied because of scaremongering by the gutter press. They seem to have created an image that stops people from helping.

The Church will be seen by how it acts, not by what it says. The Church should be doing things: putting up money for a day care centre or a hospice. Then there are the people who make up the Church, the body of the Church. We need some kind of good neighbour scheme. People may come round the hospital to talk, but what would really help is if they came round to clean the flat or do the shopping. They may be scared at first, but they must do it. I have been able to come home and stay with my mother, but the really frightening thing is to think of those with Aids who haven't any family. How are they to manage?

All the clergy I have met have treated me in a loving, compassionate way. None of them have moralised. That has brought me closer to the Church. It confirmed my faith, and made me think that their faith has got something valid, that it's not just talk. But when the Churches condemn or judge us, they are damning us with the very thing that sustains us.

The biggest tension of my life has been between my sexuality and the Church. But even now I do not believe that homosexuality is wrong. I believe it is possible to live in a "moral" relationship. A monogamous and loving relationship between two men is nothing but positive for them and the people around them. But it's clear that Mother Nature doesn't like us sleeping around. If you sleep around, you get nasty diseases. It's as simple as that.

When I recovered from the pneumonia, I went back to work, but I had to resign in the end, because it was so stressful. That I regret: it's very important to have a job for as long as you're capable of doing it. Everything was going perfectly until I got a stomach virus eight weeks ago, and I haven't been able to shift it. When I went back to the doctors I hoped it might be an ulcer, but they told me everything I didn't want to hear. That's very difficult; and sometimes I wonder what is the use of going on, to spend a year slowly dying. Sometimes I find it difficult to pray—but then I think, stick at it.

What would I say to a young homosexual? It's very difficult to educate people at that age. I never listened at that age. Knowing what I know now I would say "don't have sex, or if you must, practise safe sex". You don't catch Aids, you choose to let someone give it to you. I'd ask him if he'd like to be flat on his back in hospital being filled with toxic drugs, lose his job, spend three years slowly dying, and have to tell his parents, brothers, sisters and friends. But I still couldn't tell him homosexuality was wrong.

If I'd known then what I know now, dear me, things would have been different. A lot of the conflict between me and the

Church was of my own making. It would have been possible for me to be in a long relationship and stay in the Church, but I never talked to any priests about it. Now I have met young priests whose faith is rock hard. I should have gone and asked—there are people there.

Jim, aged 30

I was originally diagnosed antibody positive in 1982. I had the symptoms of enlarged lymph glands, sweats and fatigue, and I knew about Aids from travelling to the United States—so my doctor illegally used the American antibody test on me before it was available in this country. I remained well until 1984, when I was hospitalised with pneumonia and diagnosed with full blown Aids.

The news didn't really hit home; even my doctor wasn't sure of the implications, so as the information grew, we learned about it together. Now I'm hardened to the fact. I've had ten close friends die of Aids or Aids related illnesses since then. I've been in hospital seven times with PCP, once with cryptococcal meningitis, and once with internal KS—but having been diagnosed three and a half years ago, I'm now one of my doctor's longest living patients. It has helped that I've never had a fear of dying: once you dispel the fear of death it's much easier to cope with.

At the time I was first hospitalised, I was working as personal assistant to the managing director of a diamond company. He recognised the name of my doctor, who was becoming well known for his work with Aids patients, on the letter from the hospital and he put two and two together. He left a letter on my desk which said my services were no longer required just as he was leaving on a business trip. I had only been working for him for 11 months, so there was nothing I could do about it. I tried to find other work, but the dismissal was a problem and it would have meant lying on the medical section of every application form.

I stayed unemployed for a while, but I worked harder as a volunteer for the Terrence Higgins Trust than I ever did in full-time employment. Now I'm a paid employee of the Trust, responsible for international liaison and media resources. I also do volunteer work for the Trust as a member of a phone-counselling group, as a counsellor for Frontliners, and as a crisis intervention counsellor.

As an employee and volunteer for the Trust, and as a person with Aids, I feel that the number one issue has to be society's attitude to Aids: the stigma attached to having a terminal disease, and the added stigma of being gay.

Just before Christmas I did a TV programme for ITN. Within two days of its being shown, I was recognised in my local neighbourhood and getting all sorts of abuse in the street. One man came up and got very abusive when I was out shopping with a friend and his wife. It was very embarrassing for them. He screamed at me that I was this queer he had seen on TV that was spreading this plague. Because of the backlash, gay men may stop coming out as homosexual. Drug users also suffer a stigma. It makes it very difficult for the Trust to target the high-risk groups to educate them.

The Trust does have some difficulties with some of the religious denominations. Their teachings and the reaction to homosexuality means the Churches keep reinforcing the stigma of associating Aids always with homosexuality, and linking it with the wrath of God.

We do work directly with some like-minded religious people, who don't let their beliefs come into conflict with wanting to help. Up to 18 months ago, the gay community was as big-headed as most of the major Churches. We'd heard for so long that we had brought Aids on ourselves: why should we forgive the Churches, help them or accept help from them? There were some intelligent religious people who were getting adverse reactions from us, but they kept at it until we realised that not everyone was an enemy.

Paul, aged 42

I emigrated to the United States during the '70s with my lover, and we started a business in Texas and California. My end of it in Texas began to fail due to the oil crisis and I returned penniless to California in 1986. My lover put me out on the streets—he didn't want to deal with the financial burden.

When I was diagnosed as having ARC in September 1986 I had no medical insurance and so I had to return to England. I had applied for insurance in 1982 but it was refused because of a medical report sent by a London hospital which mentioned that I was a homosexual, although it stated that I had no medical problems. Friends paid for my airfare back to the UK, and the hospital here confirmed the diagnosis. My immunity system was shattered.

I had to find work, but it was impossible. My age, health, the fact that I'd been in the United States for 12 years all made employers very suspicious. Now I've resigned myself to the fact that I'll probably never work again. I applied for social security benefits but that was a nightmare. It took six months to sort out. The social security people have no idea how to deal with people with Aids.

I have no fixed address. I just move from one friend's house to another, sometimes sleeping on the kitchen floor just to stay warm. I applied to Kensington Council for housing, but they said I didn't meet the medical qualifications. Since my postal address is with friends in Lambeth they tried to make me start the application process all over again with Lambeth Council. I've heard horror stories about people with HIV being attacked on housing estates in the Lambeth area. The biggest problem Aids patients have once they are out of hospital is housing and care benefits. For example, I'm supposed to have a special diet which costs £22.90 a week—but I only get £17.90 for all living expenses from social security. I've borrowed over £2,000 already just to make it by.

When I was first diagnosed I was devastated, but one has the feeling that it's happening to someone else. I still haven't got it together yet. I know and accept it, but sometimes I feel so well and think it can't be me. I've been in hospital four times so far, three times with pneumonia and once suffering from distress. I'm convinced the pneumonia attacks would never have happened if I had proper housing. I also get anxiety attacks and night sweats which may mean changing the bedclothes three times a night. The doctors get us into hospital and make us well, and then the stress causes us to get sick again.

I contemplated suicide, but I decided to help other people with Aids instead, visiting, being available, and as a member of Frontliners, the support group for those who are diagnosed Aids or ARC. I get a tremendous lift out of being able to help people. Through Body Positive I met a young guy of 22 who had been diagnosed HIV-positive and was in a terrible state of worry. He was suicidal, but just by letting him talk he was able to see that things weren't so negative and he could go on with a more positive approach. I'm 42 and I've had a good life, but it's very hard to deal with when you see someone young who may only have weeks or months to live.

As a group, homosexuals are incredibly self-supporting— we're forced to be by society. And the gay population is doing more to help with the problems of Aids than people realise. Now that Aids is affecting heterosexuals, a lot of the groundwork is already done.

I was brought up in the Church of Scotland and I have always believed in God. I think there is a role for the Churches to help with Aids, but it is in giving support, not in preaching. There's so much rejection, people saying "I'm alright, Jack"—they should have more remorse. But my visits from the hospital chaplain have been very rewarding. He genuinely cared. Aids is making the Churches face up to modern reality. How can any religion say that people shouldn't use condoms?

I have no regrets about my homosexuality, although I would have taken greater care. There I totally disagree with a religious point of view. You can't make yourself homosexual or heterosexual. Aids is not a disease affecting homosexuals, it's a disease that affects mankind and it must be looked on that way.

Looking ahead, my main problem is to organise my affairs and get things into order. I need to get my belongings, over $50,000-worth, back from my ex-lover in Los Angeles. I owe so many debts to others and I don't want to leave the financial ones unresolved. But I have no means of legal representation in the US so the Terrence Higgins Trust is trying to do something through the Aids project there. My case is unusual, but most Aids patients are in a similar position in that they have overwhelming practical problems after diagnosis and no way to deal with them by themselves.

I have told a couple of members of my family that I have Aids, because every time I go into hospital I might not come out again. But I haven't told my mother. I don't want her to have to go through the experience of seeing me wilting away in agony. I've also told people I shouldn't have told, and have been rejected by them. It's devastating to be rejected by someone you care about.

William Blaney, the director of Kilmahew House drug rehabilitation centre near Glasgow, adds:

In Scotland by the end of February 1987 the number of people found to be carrying the Aids virus was 1050, the great majority of whom were drug abusers. Of that number, 11 of 16 who had been diagnosed with fully blown Aids had died. The majority of these cases are in Edinburgh and the east of Scotland, although the west, which includes Glasgow, seems to be catching up fast. It is now estimated that we will have between 400 and 700 deaths in Scotland before the end of 1989. Scotland still needs to get the message across to its drug abusing community that the sharing of needles spreads the virus and that casual sex is both sinful and suicidal.

Scotland, however, may be unusual in comparison with the rest of Britain because the drug abuser may be as young as 16 and is still very much part of his or her family. The addict may have been estranged from the family for a time, but as soon as any attempt is made to come off drugs parents and relatives respond quickly. This has also been the case with those who have been diagnosed HIV-positive and I am certain this support will continue if the young person eventually becomes ill with Aids.

Scotland may therefore have different problems in relation to Aids. The number of carriers also means 1050 families who are devastated by the news that one of their members has the virus that is seen to destroy life and destroy it very quickly. In most cases, families will turn to their local communities for help. Substitute "parishes" for community and in Scotland we have a tremendous network within the Churches, particularly through the Renew parish programme, which offers the opportunity to set up counselling and support groups. Priests and ministers are still very influential in shaping responses to crises, so they must become personally involved themselves and take the lead in encouraging initiatives.

How do you help a young addict who is HIV-positive? This is Stephen's story:

I started drinking at the age of 14 and graduated to hash by my 16th birthday. Within a few months I moved on to heroin and I loved it. It became the most important thing in my life. Prison followed, and hospital, after repeated suicide attempts. Despair came and went, but I continued injecting heroin, begging, borrowing and stealing to finance my habit, which went on for the next four years.

It was suggested that I go into Kilmahew House, Cardross, a drug rehabilitation centre. I did not like the idea one little bit, but I was sick of life and everyone was sick of me, so I went. After a month there I took stock and found to my great surprise that I enjoyed being straight. Life at long last seemed to be getting better. People told me I looked good and I certainly felt fit and happy.

Six months later, while watching television, I heard that many of the heroin addicts in Edinburgh carried the Aids virus. I was from Edinburgh and I decided to prove that not all the junkies from Edinburgh were the same, so I asked the house doctor to test me for Aids, feeling sure I was OK. Three weeks later—Bang—a positive result. God, why, why me?!! I had kicked my drug habit, I was six months clear of heroin, and I am hit with this—No kids, no wife, no sex—I might die. I will die. It's not the end, I was told; to which I thought "How the f... do you know?"

These thoughts raced through my mind at 100 mph for quite a number of months after I was told I was carrying the Aids virus. Then I started to take on board information about the virus, very slowly at first, but it started to make sense. I began to feel that I could still lead a reasonable life—but I now had to be careful.

I decided it was time to go home and see if I could cope, so I returned to my family in Edinburgh. I kept in contact with Cardross, and decided a few months later to seek readmission—but as a helper rather than as a resident. After discussions with the director I returned to help run the house and to be especially involved with those who are carrying the virus. On 7 April 1987 I celebrated two years off drugs. I have probably carried the virus longer than this, but today I am happy, I have friends and a family who love me, I am fit and healthy looking. Most of all I am at peace with myself.

Aids is not going to kill me. I am having too good a time to die. If I carry on eating right and taking some exercise, and doing what makes me happy without causing anyone else pain, I know I'll be fine. With or without the virus, I shall enjoy life, whether it's for five or 50 years. Believe me, Aids is not the end.

8 | Women with Aids

Janine Railton
Aids promotion officer for the
Riverside Health Unit

Many women have come forward since the introduction of the HIV antibody test, and particularly since the enormous amount of media coverage on Aids in recent months. Very few of these women have tested positive. Several reasons why so many have requested the test spring to mind: they may be more health conscious than men; they may have more sexual partners than is generally recognised; they may be afraid of their sexuality; or they may be confronting the Aids problem more readily than men. The last explanation is supported by an examination of the reasons women give for taking the test. Many women attend the sexually transmitted disease clinic for HIV testing because their past or present sexual partners were bisexual or drug abusers. What we do not know is whether these women are telling the truth, or fabricating a reason for fear of having the test refused. On the other hand, Asian and West Indian women may feel that Aids is not an issue for them as they come from very close-knit family groups. But this needs to be challenged, since other sexually transmitted diseases have been widely found in these groups.

A traumatic experience

It is not uncommon for women in stable relationships to attend the clinic for an HIV test, some of whom are considering pregnancy or who may have recently discovered they are pregnant. The fact that women are taking the HIV test before becoming pregnant supports the theory that they are becoming more health conscious and they are taking the media information campaign on Aids seriously. Some women attending the clinic in early pregnancy are unsure of their feelings about their condition or the baby, but are adamant that if the test should prove positive they would definitely have a termination. In reality, termination for a woman with HIV infection is a very traumatic experience. Burdened already with the knowledge that she has an almost certainly fatal disease, she must cope with the fact that she may have transmitted it to her unborn infant. With the termination goes almost certainly her last chance at motherhood, something that few women would wish to miss.

There have been several cases of women with the virus becoming pregnant. Of 25 women who attend St Stephen's Hospital and Westminster Hospital at the time of writing, seven have been pregnant. Three babies have been delivered, one is due, two pregnancies were terminated and one was ectopic. Whether or not the woman chooses termination, the guilt is the same: that for ending the pregnancy or for having transmitted the virus to a child. I have also known two women who were antibody negative, with HIV-positive partners, who became pregnant. Both women miscarried while attempting to make the decision about termination, and both were relieved at having the onus for the decision taken away from them. In both cases, the women themselves have remained free of HIV infection.

53

I have also seen couples where the man was HIV-positive and the woman uninfected who would like to have a family. The male partner is well and may remain so for a long time, but the risk of transmitting the virus is too great for them to consider starting a family. These women would like to be able to adopt, or be recipients of artificial insemination by anonymous donor. They would like to remain with their partner but experience the joy of bringing up a child. To these women, that society does not allow them either option seems like a punishment to them for loving a man who is HIV-positive.

Faced with grief

Women with the virus who have continued with the pregnancy and then lost a child from Aids have suffered immense grief. In many cases a mother will only learn that she herself has the virus when the child is born showing signs of immunodeficiency. She must come to terms at the same time with being infected with HIV, and with the child's imminent death from the virus. If a woman gives birth to a baby with Aids, who will look after it? Who will die first? Families and friends of children with HIV have been afraid to touch them, and these children, who like any others need to be cuddled and loved, have been left isolated and uncared for. Our society is very cruel. The community can be very hard on adults with Aids, but even harder on children who are unable to fight for themselves.

I have been astounded by the inner strength of women who have learnt that they are antibody positive, especially those who have acquired the virus through blood transfusion or from their partners. They draw on extraordinary resources to fight the virus in a society that still considers Aids to be a gay man's disease. One woman who entered a London hospital had acquired the virus abroad from a blood transfusion after the birth of her child. The family returned to England when her health inexplicably deteriorated. Her husband rarely visited her and he kept the child away. I have never seen anyone who wanted to hold on to her life so badly. She fought Aids until the very last minute in almost complete isolation.

Closely guarded secret

Because there are so few women with the virus, there is little fellowship with others in the same position, and they feel isolated. There are few heterosexual men who are infected with whom to form new relationships. They may have little in common with gay men. These women are also afraid of mixing with their own friends in case they break down and tell someone. Women who are HIV-infected must choose whether to be open about it or keep it a closely guarded secret. In my experience, most women choose the latter option. Women's social and work lives tend to overlap more than those of men, so that keeping the information confidential among a few is more difficult. For many women, who have always been very open about their feelings, this can be an enormous strain. Nevertheless, this same openness can be an advantage for these women when working with a counsellor or other carers. While men have been taught to keep a "stiff upper lip", women have traditionally been allowed to have "a good old-fashioned cry", and this can make the role of caring for them much easier.

Prostitution and drugs

Because of the risk of catching sexually transmitted diseases other than Aids, many prostitutes have taken the precaution of insisting that their clients use condoms for many years. Health education has reached many of them, but not all: some men will pay a prostitute more to have sex without a condom, and, since sex for money is the aim and many prostitutes are still controlled by pimps, the prostitute's fear of the pimp may well outweigh her fear of a sexually transmitted disease. Prostitutes who are supporting a drug habit may be even less concerned about the risk of acquiring or transmitting the Aids virus. As yet, few prostitutes in this country are known to have HIV infection.

In considering prostitution, it is easy to forget that also exists among men. Male prostitutes may or may not be heterosexuals, and may themselves have girlfriends, and their clients are often married men who are closet gays. One wonders how many of these men have acquired the virus and passed it on to their wives.

Few women as a percentage of the total attending clinics for HIV testing are proving to be antibody positive. But the UK figures for heterosexually transmitted Aids are now similar to those for homosexual men three years ago. It is important that we do not become complacent, thinking that it really isn't our problem. We do not know the full scale of what is to come and the accuracy of our estimates will only be evaluated when it is too late. The women who are attending clinics, questioning their partners, and changing their sexual behaviour and lifestyles are taking responsibility for their own health and setting the example we should all be following. It is the only way to combat this killer virus.

PART III | Aids and the Christian family

9 The Christian family and the media

Douglas Brown

Freelance journalist, formerly BBC religious affairs correspondent

Aids and the way the media has dealt with it: what effect have all those column inches and hours of air time had on the family? To attempt to answer that question is a formidable undertaking. Aids unites and divides. There can be few families, Christian or otherwise, that do not share the fear of one of their number becoming infected by the sickness for which there is no cure, particularly parents for their children. But the reaction to the media coverage between Christians and non-Christians reflects as few things have done in recent times the divisions between those motivated by religious conviction and those who reject it. This is shown above all by the emphasis on ways of preventing the disease.

Christians argue that the virtue of chastity consistently taught by their faith is the sure preventative against Aids. Non-Christians put the emphasis on the physical, the mechanical precautions that should be taken by a society that assumes non-chastity almost as a way of life. This attitude is the one, by and large, that has been reflected by most of the media and by the government campaign. It is, to put it bluntly, the tension between chastity and the condom.

The failure of the media

Christians, of course, are not of one mind over matters sexual. Contraception, a practice permitted by most of the Churches of the Reformation, is officially rejected by Roman Catholicism. There are bound, therefore, to be differences in the strength of reaction to the secular emphasis on contraceptive measures to prevent Aids between those Roman Catholics who strictly adhere to the teaching of the Church and the majority of non-Catholics. Homosexual practice is strictly forbidden by Vatican decree, an attitude shared by many fundamentalist Protestants. Other Churches react in less prescriptive ways, with attitudes seen by some fellow Christians as permissive and by others as compassionate. But what unites is far stronger than what

59

divides, and Christians are at one over the teaching of virginity for the unmarried, continence for the widowed, loyalty to the husband and wife for the married. It is the failure of so much of the secular media to reflect this, both as the ideal of sexual behaviour and as a way of containing the Aids epidemic, that Christians by and large have found so offensive, particularly parents.

The precautions of a faithful marriage

So vast has the output on Aids been of late that it would be folly to make unqualified statements on the media overall. No one person could read every column inch that has been printed or watch or listen to every minute of broadcasting. But, during the special Aids week on television, I saw nearly all the output and in only one short programme found any emphasis on abstention from intercourse outside marriage as a way of containing the disease. What may well remain vividly in the minds of millions of viewers were the several demonstrations of fitting a condom on a plastic penis, something which many parents watching with their children must have found both acutely embarrassing, to put it mildly, and singularly calculated to defeat the efforts of those trying to bring up their sons and daughters in the virtue of Christian chastity.

Certainly no-one can be excused for not knowing all there is to know clinically about Aids after seven days of such intensive coverage especially from the BBC. Some of it was very sophisticated, including, for instance, the *Horizon* programme on the treatment of Aids; the feature that looked at the way the media in other countries were warning of the hazards; the late-night phone-ins; the answers to young people's questions; the *QED* biological guide; the erudite *Science on 3*. But all the time the emphasis was on "playing safe". It was summed up in a blurb in the *Radio Times* for one of the nightly series on "Facing up to Aids": "By taking a few precautions and practising safer sex people can continue to share loving relations." What kind of loving relations? What of the precautions of a faithful marriage? Even *Heart of the Matter*, which might have been expected to show a BBC nod in the direction of traditional teaching chose, perhaps with an eye on the ratings, to deal with homosexuals and the prejudices being shown towards them with the advent of Aids.

ITV coverage was less copious, but like that of the BBC left no-one in any doubt of the dangers of Aids—what to do if

60

you think you've got it, what prospects there are of a cure being found, the inevitable glimpse of the gay community and, of course, the ubiquitous condom. But I saw no-one on either network give a straightforward explanation of Christian teaching on sex. And Christian thinkers on moral issues are among the best broadcasters in the business.

Hundreds of words of slush

And so to what our American cousins call the "print media". If we have misgivings about the television and radio approach to Aids, they are as nothing compared to those regarding the popular press, the mass-circulation tabloids. They have exceeded themselves in sensationalism and vulgarity, in trivialising and insensitivity. The *News of the World* splashed this headline across two pages: "I wanted to give my wife a baby. Instead I gave her Aids." The story began with "Peter wanted to give his pretty wife Angela a baby to make their happy marriage complete—but instead he gave her Aids and turned their dream into a nightmare". No, Peter was not a rake. The unfortunate young man was a haemophiliac who caught the disease through routine treatment. The tragic circumstances of their life were told in hundreds of words of unmitigated slush.

"Torment of the tragic rent boy" was the headline over a *Mirror* story about male prostitutes which began: "Alex is one of 18 tragic 'rent boys' who have become a deadly menace to their customers—because they have Aids." A few sentences later; "But he is still plying his deadly trade. And at the moment it seems that society is powerless to stop him." And a picture of a young man with the caption: "For sale: a rent boy waits for a customer." "Aids squad spacemen collect dead teacher" was the *Sun* headline over the story of the collection by policemen in protective clothing of the HIV-infected teacher who had committed suicide. With, of course, a picture of the "space squad" in action with the coffin. "Children of the Damned", in type as big as any known to the trade, was the way the *Daily Star* introduced a so-called special on children born to parents with Aids, plus a picture of baby in cot. And, for good measure, under the tag "world exclusive", an interview with a young mother, a former heroin addict now waiting to see if she has passed on the virus to her child. "I felt like a leper", screamed the headline and "Living a nightmare" began the caption under a picture of mother, father and baby.

Again under the predictable "exclusive" tag, inch-high

headlines in the *Sunday Express* announced "Aids 'made in lab' shock" and the story began, "The killer Aids virus was artificially created by American scientists during laboratory experiments which went disastrously wrong—and a massive cover-up has kept the secret from the world until today. That is the sensational claim made independently by three international experts—and they reject the widely-held belief that Aids originated after an African green monkey bit a man." "Sensational claim." But what of the proof? What, indeed!

Trivialising and sensationalising the crisis

But the *Sun*, none other, in a page feature complete with anatomical picture under the heading: "Have you got Aids: 10 ways to find out" also had a subheading: "10 ways to avoid catching it" which ended with these remarkable words: "The message: don't sleep around, stay with a faithful, safe and reliable partner." A wife, for instance? Other choice headlines have included: "Hit show that is dying of Aids"; "Double curse of the Aids Plague City" (no, not San Francisco but Edinburgh); "How Aids is destroying New York's Trendy Set"; and many more in similar vein.

An old friend of mine in a senior position in the newsroom of a highly responsible organisation told me that they had followed up over the months most of the Aids stories in the mass-circulation tabloids. They found so many of them either groundless or hyped-up from the flimsiest of evidence that they no longer bothered even to check on them. I am not alleging that the stories I have quoted are not based on fact. But here we have journals that go into millions of homes trivialising and sensationalising the Aids crisis, and constantly debasing the sexual dimension for a readership largely untrained to be discerning and critical of media coverage. Moreover, children are now being assailed by the disturbing juxtaposition of sex, disease and death instead of the ideal that sex is an expression of love, joy and procreation.

The quality papers

So, then, to the serious daily and Sunday papers. Their coverage, on the whole, has been responsible, aware and extensive. I particularly liked the restrained way *The Independent* covered the issue of euthanasia in Holland, the story itself a sober reminder of a problem that may soon exercise the minds of many doctors and moralists and become a major pastoral challenge to the Churches. From the same stable came a particular careful piece on avoiding promiscuity abroad, above all in Africa where the virus is already rampant in the sub-Saharan areas.

The Times, back in July 1983 under the heading "Aids is here", may have been the first of the quality newspapers to alert the public of this country to the full significance of the epidemic, with a full-page article running into more than 3,000 words on all its alarming aspects. It concluded by quoting Michael Adler, professor of genito-urinary medicine at the Middlesex Hospital, saying: "I can't believe we're going to have an unsolved problem for more than two years." That Professor Adler was over-optimistic is sadly all-too-apparent, but in all this wide-ranging article there was no hint of the moral aspects of the disease, nothing to point to the fact that Christian teaching could be the way to eliminate it.

The Times followed this article a few weeks later with a slight editorial nod in the direction of Christian teaching. "The Aids risk is attendant on sexual promiscuity, and on intravenous drug abuse or infected instruments. Avoid those forms of behaviour and the risk of contracting Aids is reduced almost to vanishing point in any society that observes standard rules of personal and medical hygiene. If the methods of Hippocrates let us down, the methods of Savonarola are available for our protection." But why Savonarola? Isn't what counts above all the teaching of Jesus and St Paul? And would Savonarola's high-pressure ranting against promiscuity be taken any more seriously today than by the 15th-century Florentines? Isn't something more incisive needed?

As far back as the end of 1985 the religious affairs correspondent of *The Times*, Clifford Longley, began his weekly article with the timely assertion that the Christian Churches, acting as guardians of sexual morality, could become the government's most important allies in the campaign for education against Aids. He ended: "The issue for churchmen now is whether they can devise a programme of public education themselves that would stand a reasonable chance of changing people's moral attitudes and behaviour in favour of chastity." Some would say that the issue, 19 months later, is very much the same.

But what leading churchmen have had to say has been widely and carefully reported in the quality press. None more so than one of the clearest and most challenging voices of them all,

63

Archbishop Thomas Winning of Glasgow. However commendable the intentions of government and television companies, he said, their approach seemed founded on certain assumptions that could not go unquestioned. He went on: "The ruthless cynicism which suggests that unbridled sexual acivity is not only inevitable but the normal way that people act at present contains a pessimistic and patronising view of human nature which many justifiably resent and reject. The Christian teaching of fidelity within marriage and chastity outside it corresponded to the best medical advice on "safe sex". The archbishop called for "an altogether more wholesome attitude on the part of the media".

No other churchman in this country has so sharply and unequivocally condemned media coverage and overall attitudes than Archbishop Winning. Others have sought to make similar points, but have so often hedged them around with verbal placebos that the impact has been blunted. A pamphlet from the Church of England's Board for Social Responsibility was accused by *The Independent's* religious affairs correspondent, Andrew Brown, of ducking the issue and concentrating on those already suffering from the disease. There followed a quote from the pamphlet: "We know enough to prevent the further spread of the disease . . . the problem lies in . . . identifying carriers and . . . ensuring that their contacts with others, sexual or otherwise, are such that the virus is not transmitted." Andrew Brown added: "There are no details of how this might be done. If you thought the Board for Social Responsibility would take words like chastity or fidelity into its mouth, you thought wrong." Curiously, it was an ex-B movie actor who coined the sharpest slogan of them all: "You don't teach how to do it, but that you don't do it," President Reagan told American doctors.

Selling people short

The government's own campaign must not be overlooked, for you would expect from it an element of the ethical and moral. But no. The shock approach—Aids kills—in the disturbing but unspecific 40-second tombstone film was followed by an information leaflet delivered to households on how to avoid Aids with the words: "It is safest to stick to one partner." Of course it is, but no word on Christian marriage. Yet some of the leaders of all the parties are fond of reminding us that we are still a Christian country, and Parliament begins its daily sessions with prayer.

What, then, of the church papers? One, the Roman Catholic *Universe*, has launched a campaign which reflects Archbishop Winning, saying in a leaflet aimed particularly at the 15–25 age-group, but applicable to all, that the present publicity campaign sells people short, especially the young, and urges everyone to rule out sex before marriage and choose a lifelong partner who shares your moral convictions. Some 200,000 of these leaflets have been distributed in Catholic parishes and elsewhere.

The other church papers have not sold their readers short. *The Church Times* has had two careful editorials reflecting compassion towards people with Aids and emphasising Christian teaching. Outstanding among *Catholic Herald* articles was one from Joyce Poole, a Catholic general practitioner, which concluded: "The dilemma of the bishops on the Aids problem insofar as it springs from the Church's stand on contraception may seem to us a dilemma of unreality. A kind of emperor's new clothes situation. I share the anxiety of some, perhaps many, Catholic doctors that if the Church continues to make pronouncements about sexual behaviour which disregard reality, that it will be in danger of losing credence and authority on other issues at the centre of our faith and precious to us all."

The quality weeklies have, on the whole, reflected in more leisurely and cerebral manner the argument patterns of the serious daily papers, apart from *The Tablet*, which has sought to reconcile the teaching of the Church with the realities of the situation.

Intellectual wrestling

Not that the weeklies always resist twisting issues for the sake of sensationalism, just like the tabloids they are so often at pains to scorn. Piers Paul Read, for instance, in a *Spectator* article headed "Sex and Sin" unjustifiably smears the *Times* article by Cardinal Hume reprinted in this volume. In this carefully-worded contribution, the cardinal did in fact write that something more radical was called for than the scourging of other people's vices, but unequivocally made the point that the full expression of love was reserved for husband and wife. According to Mr Read, the cardinal suggested "no more than that 'the Judaeo-Christian heritage of moral values still has much to offer contemporary society' ". The cardinal did much more. He said: "The Roman Catholic Church cannot be expected to lend support to any measures which tacitly accept, even if they don't encourage, sexual activity outside marriage".

Amid all the intellectual wrestling in the secular weeklies, I have only space for one more example. It was from Dr Anthony Clare in *The Listener*'s centrepiece. His conclusion is one that no-one who pays any service at all to the Christian dimension can afford to ignore, "Today", says Anthony Clare, "doctors may join clergymen in calling for sexual restraint, monogamy, even chastity. But should there be a breakthrough in control of the virus, many doctors would vacate the pulpit as quickly as they occupied it. This is another lesson to be learned from a study of medical history and it is a lesson that society would do well to ponder."

Among the tens of thousands of words I've read for this article, these impressed me most of all, getting as they do to the heart of the challenge of Aids to the Christian Churches, the family and the media alike. Once Aids can be cured or prevented or both, will there be an overnight return to the permissive society?

10 The retreat from the '60s: a mother's point of view

Alison Skelton
Novelist and mother

My children were in primary school when I first heard of the disease we now call Aids. It hadn't even a name then, and its nature was not yet defined. It was merely an oddity puzzling doctors in America; a footnote in *Time* magazine. Nothing could have seemed more remote to the small Highland community into which my children were born.

Three years later, on a visit to New York, I found the homosexual communities of Greenwich Village and the Fire Island beaches tense with awareness of Aids. No longer a medical curiosity, it was, within that segment of society, already seen as a growing threat. Aids had become the gay plague. Though other affected groups were already known, it was still possible, outside the gay community, to regard it with some sanguinity.

Today, no-one can afford that selfish luxury. In less than a decade Aids has become a serious threat to the health of people in all countries and all communities. In the same few years, my children have grown to the edge of adulthood. They are the first "Aids generation". What do we, as parents, say and do to help them meet this alarming new challenge?

As a practising Catholic, I am of course presented with one solution of unnerving simplicity: obey the dictates of the Church. Premarital chastity, post-marital fidelity, an avoidance of hard drugs and the rejection of proscribed sexual activities; rarely have ecclesiastical and medical advice meshed so beautifully. But nothing is ever so simple as that. The Church has not been the only influence upon sexual mores in recent times; indeed it has fought a defensive battle, some would say an obstructive one, against the changes of the sexual revolution. There lies the core of my discomfort with the entire question of Aids and morality.

Like many parents today, I am a child of the '60s. My generation experienced more freedom and less fear in sexual matters than any before. Venereal diseases were readily treatable, pregnancy was subject to the control of effective contraception, and childbirth itself had been made much safer. The external limits on sexuality that had served as controls on our parents' behaviour were largely gone. All that remained were religious strictures that seemed to many out-dated and which were under attack by a new moral code, based heavily upon Freud. In the received wisdom of the day sex was not only natural and wholesome, but essential to our well-being. The bogey-man of our youth was not the dangers inherent in the free expression of sexuality, but those inherent in its repression.

The legacy of "free love"

Even before Aids, however, disquiet was expressed by today's young over the philosophies of that freer era. Each generation rejects something of the one before, perhaps because it lives to see the realities that emerged from its predecessor's dreams. The experimentation during the '60s with hallucinogens has been judged by its legacy of heroin and cocaine addiction. The "free love" revolution bequeathed soaring divorce rates and broken families. And now there is this eerie plague—small wonder if the superstitious see it as the act of an avenging (though hardly Christian) God. The sins of the fathers. . . . It would not be surprising if our children held us to blame.

How then can we presume to address them in a tone of

parental authority and experience, without descending into unforgiveable hypocrisy? How can we lecture them on the need for moral restraint when we had precious little ourselves? We stand besieged in a castle built on the sand of our own careless youth.

Aids has undoubtedly altered the moral strictures I would lay before my children. The Church's rulings on sexual matters, which I once regarded as at best an ideal I did not really expect them to attain and at worst an unreasonable shackling that might do more harm than good, now appear to offer their greatest safety. One might rejoice in this meek return to the fold, but there is no true virtue in a decision based on fear. Regardless, the more practical issue remains: will they obey such strictures anyhow? And if they do, how will they manage the difficult task of finding partners and making successful marriages in the new social climate that will result?

Earlier eras demanded greater chastity from young people, but in such eras parental authority was strong and the choice of a marriage partner often a family matter in which adult judgment struck a sober balance with youthful romance. Today's young people are left much more alone to make perhaps the most serious decision of their lives. Naivety and romantic innocence do not seem likely to make the choosing easier. I look ahead uneasily to a generation of young, rather desperate marriages, partnerships against the threat of a sexually dangerous world. Fear is not a rock upon which to found the families of the future.

Faced with our own sorry history

When a 16-year-old says to me, resignedly, "it might have been better if the '60s never happened", (the '60s being his catch-phrase for all the social changes of the era) it is a chilling judgment on my generation's contribution to the world. What can I answer?

What was gained from the freedoms of our youth, now about to be denied our children? Sexual experimentation did not bring about the more mature or more stable relationships that might have been hoped for. Were that so, our marriages should be sound and steady and our divorce rate plummetting rather than soaring. Much weight was placed upon the importance of sexual compatibility in the foundations of a marriage. But such physical communion is not a constant. Happy lovers are radically changed by the arrival of children, the loss of a job, a death in the family. A good sexual relationship is laboriously built and subject to constant adjustment; it is not just a happy find in the lottery of the singles bar.

Faced with our own sorry history, it is all too easy to say to our children, "It wasn't worth it; you're missing nothing anyhow". But such advice sounds pompous at best. "*We* found out everything for ourselves, now you must take our word for it, and do not what we did but what we tell you to do." If I were 16, that wouldn't appeal much to me.

Love deeper than passion

I think we must be more honest. Yes. It is thoroughly unfair. But there are no guarantees for any generation. Our parents faced economic depression and war. We grew up under the shadow of Hiroshima. You have Aids. And at the moment, it doesn't look like that is going to change. It simply must be dealt with and "use a condom and do what you will" is hardly a solution. There is no such thing as safe casual sex, only *safer* sex, and when the losing ticket is death it is a lottery no one seriously wishes to play. Besides, what kind of lovemaking are we imagining; armouring ourselves against the beloved, filled with fear and distrust and suspicion over past follies unrevealed? Is simple sensation worth all that?

No. The days of sensation for its own sake are done. The pace must slow. Love must return to the love act, and love is a deeper, more thoughtful thing than passion. Courtship must become just that, not simply a bargaining ground in which promises of affection are rewarded with physical treats.

Some young people, particularly young women, might welcome the change. I was certainly aware of '60s girls who longed wistfully for a reason to say no, when all the old reasons were gone. Today, a more liberated young woman might choose to say, "No, my body is my own. It always will be. Even when I'm married. No one will exercise rights over it other than me."

Young men, too, might find relief from the relentless pressure to achieve sexual experience before they are ready for it or even desire it. They too have been caught in a trap that demanded overt sexuality as a proof of some idea of maturity. I found it most ironic that on a recent television discussion about Aids the young man who honestly, if bashfully, admitted he was yet a virgin, was subjected to instantaneous laughter and humiliation from the supposedly serious and concerned audience (and interviewer!) in the studio.

I would like to see young men confident enough to say, "Yes, I'm male. I've got the same kind of body as the rest of you. I don't really have to do anything to prove it." After all, isn't it a little strange that sex, which is one of the few of our many talents that takes nothing special in the way of intelligence or physical ability—after all, just about *everyone* can do it— should so long have loomed so important in our assessment of each other?

Perhaps this adolescent obsession will fade with the generation that birthed it. We '60s people were a very adolescent generation, obsessed with youth itself. And now we are growing old and finding ourselves sternly regarded by our own children. Still, before we retire shame-facedly from the scene, let us lay before those children our few achievements.

The fine lost art of fidelity

We had extraordinary freedom. Out of freedom came a generosity of spirit that engendered tolerance and compassion. It was in our era that homosexual love was accorded a share of the dignity due to all love. It was in our era that young unwed mothers began to feel they might keep and love their children rather than bear them in secret and shame and give them up to others. There was a disdain of hypocrisy and a softening of the traditional boundaries between the sexes that provided new outlets for the "masculine" traits of women and the "feminine" traits of men. A new closer relationship developed between fathers and small children, from the moment of childbirth onwards. Childbirth itself became a celebration of family life. It wasn't all bad.

And so, I would say to my children, "It's over. You cannot live as we did. You will be required to exert more self-discipline, more self-denial. You will need patience and restraint, rarely virtues of the young. You will have to be courageous, even to seek love. You will gain, if you are honest, in personal integrity and in the fine lost art of fidelity. But do not, if you can help it, lose the gentle spirit of our age. Let us not go back to a world in which homosexuals are hounded and harried and children born out of wedlock bear the old stigma of bastardy. Let us not return to all that secrecy and shame. Let us achieve, if we can, a new purity without descending into a new puritan age."

70

11 | Aids and morality

Jack Dominian

Consultant psychiatrist at the
Central Middlesex Hospital, London

I find Aids all the more distressing because the Christian
community is largely unprepared to offer a convincing response,
in terms of sexual morality, to the challenge posed by this
terrible disease. To advocate abstinence from sex before marriage
and faithfulness within it is to proclaim the traditional Christian
teaching. But the world of today no longer accepts this teaching as
a given. A case has to be made for it. In my travels both at home
and abroad, I find a singular absence of such a convincing case.
And yet the catastrophe of Aids is challenging us urgently to
present the Christian teaching in its most persuasive light.

During the last quarter of a century, there has been a marked
alteration in sexual and marital behaviour without an equivalent
Christian reassessment. Two thousand years of Christianity
have attuned us to link sexuality primarily with one objective:
procreation. This has led to a morality largely based on biology,
centred on the fusion of sperm and ovum and the appropriate
conditions for bringing this about. The insufficiency of such an
outlook has always been obvious but the biological
underpinning of sexual morality was shattered, with huge social
implications, when the separation of procreation and
intercourse became easy and widespread. This happened in the
early '60s and the consequences have been dramatic.

Non-procreative

Increasingly, throughout the world today, most marital
intercourse is non-procreative. Ninety-nine per cent of sexual
activity within marriage is knowingly and deliberately non-
procreative, whatever the means of birth control which are
used. So Christianity is faced with a new situation which is
likely to remain with us permanently.

Some people may say that I exaggerate the extent to which
Christianity has linked sex and procreation. Surely, they may ask,
other purposes of sexual intercourse have been admitted:
especially, indeed, the strengthening of the love between the
couple. Sadly, however, this has yet to be fully explored and

71

understood. Very little has been written about it. As far as the Roman Catholic Church is concerned, the advances of the second Vatican Council on the meaning of sexual intercourse within marriage have largely been ignored because of the heated debate over *Humanae Vitae*.

Christianity can learn from the world in its attitude to sexuality. The world has widely sanctioned the goodness of sexual activity. This Christianity can unequivocally accept. Now is the time for Christians to disclaim any negative view of sexual intercourse. They can proclaim loud and clear that it is one of the most precious gifts of the Creator, with a richness of meaning that goes far beyond the biological.

The world has also gone far to break the link between sex and biology through widespread birth regulation. This has been a source of considerable anxiety to the Christian community, particularly the Roman Catholic Church. This is not the place to return to the contraceptive controversy. It is the place, however, to assert categorically that what has to be considered is men and women as persons, and the link between them, based on love, rather than biological functions.

Lastly, Christianity can learn from the significant advances which the world has made during the last quarter of a century in understanding the formation and preservation of human bonding. The importance of sex as a basis both for mutual attraction and for the subsequent maintenance of marriage is receiving increasing attention particularly in psychological circles. This personal dimension of human sexuality has to be the foundation of the emerging morality.

Christianity rightly considers the family of enormous significance. Yet families are founded on the man-woman relationship which precedes the arrival of children, is responsible for their care and nurture, and survives several decades after their departure. No equivalent effort has been made to understand and service this relationship. It has taken large-scale marital breakdown to make us realise how much spouses in their own right need help and support.

The proper place of courtship

Despite appearances to the contrary, the intense natural power of sexuality is not primarily directed towards pleasure or procreation, but towards bond formation and thereafter the maintenance of the bond formed. In the second chapter of Genesis God affirms: "It is not right that man should be alone."

At the heart of the mystery of creation is relationship, and a loving relationship between man and woman is fundamental. A Trinitarian faith that believes in the mystery of the divine persons in relationships of love should not find the revelation surprising.

Thus Christianity should have no problem in proclaiming sexuality to be that force which impels men and women towards the formation and maintenance of an exclusive relationship. In practice when a man and a woman are attracted towards each other, the impulse is towards sexual intercourse to complete the bonding process. But there is a need for clarity here. The desire to have sexual intercourse in order to become one is part of the process of personal bonding; its significance cannot be confined to physical orgasm. Premarital promiscuity distorts the meaning of sexual attraction. The man or woman who seeks bodily pleasure in the absence of personal encounter is dehumanising all that sexual attraction seeks to achieve and the body can rebel against such treatment through venereal disease or cancer or both.

What our society needs to restore is the proper place of courtship. This phase ensures that sexual attraction acts as a stimulus for deepening awareness of each other as persons.

Some may say that premarital cohabitation achieves precisely this. Certainly most living together on a basis which is mostly exclusive and faithful is not promiscuity and should not be placed in that category. It is nevertheless sexual intercourse outside marriage. Here some would argue that the issue is not sexual morality but the nomenclature of marriage. At one period in the history of the Church such exclusive, faithful and committed relationships sealed with sexual intercourse were regarded to be valid marriages, and some sociologists today regard cohabitation as part of marriage. Nevertheless, the stability of marriage is so important that it should be given every support, and the greatest possible strength is conferred by a public declaration.

Sustaining the bond

Once a permanent bond called marriage is established, modern health care combined with social change has reduced the biological link between intercourse and procreation to a minimum. What needs to be expanded enormously is our understanding of the role of intercourse in maintaining the husband-wife relationship for the growth and nurture in love of

73

the children. I have written extensively about this elsewhere. The findings of psychology have proved beyond question the need for children to be brought up by parents whose marriages are secure. We are being made increasingly aware of the tremendous damage inflicted on families by an unstable or broken marriage.

Intercourse is primarily concerned with the formation and maintenance of human bonds. When such a bond exists, extramarital intercourse is a violation of that relationship of love and threatens it, as well as causing immense pain. As repeated surveys have shown, society may hesitate to condemn premarital intercourse, but has no such reservation in condemning adultery.

As always when Christian teaching is authentic, the advocacy of faithfulness and premarital chastity does not inhibit but proclaims and assists human integrity. Aids has drawn our attention to the need to avoid promiscuity, but we have to go far more deeply into the implications. At its simplest level, promiscuity is the pursuit of sexual pleasure, and in considering the matter many go no further. All of us working in the field of human relationships know that there is much more to it than that.

Safeguards for the family

The man or woman who pursues sexual contacts relentlessly is often a deeply hurt and wounded human being who is incapable of forming stable loving relationships. These vulnerable people have often had very disturbed childhoods. The current large-scale marital instability is producing a vicious circle, for in turn the wounded children of such marriages are the potential alcoholics, drug addicts, disordered personalities, young offenders and sexual deviants of the future. The Aids crisis must make us look more deeply at the instability of family life in the West.

Christian awareness in the field of sexuality and marriage has greatly increased, but there is still need for much more study. Against a background of such neglect, sexual abuse and marital breakdown are taking a severe toll. The arrival of Aids is a reminder of the need to give priority to finding new ways of proclaiming the truth about sexual conduct and safeguarding the family, the fundamental human unit. For this, we need thought, funding and research. I have made such pleas repeatedly over the last 25 years and I am extremely sad that the occasion of a fresh call should be the potential disaster of Aids. If catastrophe is to be avoided and effective progress in sexual and marital matters to be made, an enormous effort is needed and I appeal to everyone to make it. The world is hungry for the message.

But we must avoid simplistic solutions. Faced with the crisis of Aids it is urgent and imperative that a sexual and marital morality based not on fear but on personal love should be established in the Christian community. St John makes it clear that fear and love are not compatible. In proclaiming love Christianity must not only advocate discipline and self-control, but also search the hearts and minds of ordinary people for the contemporary meaning of sexuality and marriage. We need to take all that is best in our tradition and combine it with the most recent advances made by the psychological sciences in understanding human nature, so as to present it anew.

© *The Tablet*, 10 January 1987

PART IV | Theologians reflect

12 | Because they suffer

Gareth Moore OP
Dominican friar at Blackfriars, Oxford

There is one saying of Jesus that unites both Old and New Testaments:

> You shall love the Lord your God with all your heart, and with all your soul, and with all your mind. This is the great and first commandment. And a second is like it: you shall love your neighbour as yourself. On these two commandments depend all the law and the prophets[1].

If we are to love our neighbour as ourselves, this certainly means doing all we can to meet the needs of our neighbours who are sick and dying. And if we should ask, "but who is our neighbour?", we need only turn to the parable of the Good Samaritan for an answer[2].

If we need any more convincing, there is another famous teaching of Jesus. In St Matthew's gospel, Jesus's final discourse to the disciples is about the Last Judgment. Then it will be, he says, as when a shepherd separates the sheep from the goats. The sheep, those who have done good, will enter the kingdom to enjoy eternal life, while the goats will go to eternal punishment in the fire prepared for the devil and his angels[3]. And the criterion by which all will be judged is whether they have ministered to Christ in the person of the needy:

> Then the King will say to those at his right hand: "Come, O blessed of my Father, inherit the Kingdom prepared for you from the foundation of the world; for I was hungry and you gave me drink, I was a stranger and you welcomed me, I was naked and you clothed me, I was sick and you visited me, I was in prison and you came to me. . . . As you did it to one of the least of these my brethren, you did it to me"[4].

In fact, Christians have never needed much convincing about this. In Christianity, ministering to those in need and tending the sick has always been prominent.

The first and only thing we have to know about Aids sufferers is that many of them are dying. Even if they are not in immediate danger, they must come to terms with death as imminent, often at a very young age. This fact alone makes it

79

natural, as a matter of course, for the Church to make itself available to give what help it can to Aids sufferers who need it. We are followers to him who said: "I came that they may have life, and have it abundantly"[5], and we recognise that our end and the end of all human beings, the mystery that we call God, is life itself. This may involve helping people with Aids to take care of their material needs and providing companionship for them. It will certainly involve helping them to face death. As members of the Church have been prepared to give of themselves to help the victims of plagues throughout history, often endangering themselves in the process, as they have always been prepared to help the sick and the dying, so we can and should be confident that the Church will do so again in this case.

But . . . There are no buts. Some people, though, have wanted to suggest that there are. They might want to say that Aids is different because those who suffer from it are by and large not innocent victims. There are those who get it through no fault of their own—haemophiliacs, babies, faithful wives infected by faithless husbands—but mostly you get Aids by sinning. It is prostitutes and their clients who get it; and those clients include married and therefore adulterous men. It is drug addicts who get it, those who have abused and destroyed the body God has given them; and of course, most of all, gay men. It is these last above all who have given Aids a bad name, have turned it into the wrath of God, a punishment for flouting the divine and natural law. For we know that the law condemns to death people who do such things[6].

It is implied that these people do not deserve our sympathy and that we ought to be on God's side and join in the condemnation. Aids sufferers have put themselves beyond the pale, and they are to be rebuked rather than helped. We can rejoice in the justice of God. By this argument, our love of God dispenses us from the requirement to love our neighbour.

The suffering of the psalmists

This, of course, is wrong. The short answer to it is that when Jesus says we are to love our neighbour as ourselves, he does not add: provided he is no sinner. When he tells us to go to those in prison, he does not say that it is only to the innocent and the wrongly condemned that we are to show the love of God. Simply, those who are being punished, for whatever reason, are entitled to our care not *in spite of* their crimes, but *because of* their suffering. Their crimes are irrelevant. Neither does Jesus bid us to visit the sick provided that they are "innocent victims."

80

Our job, always and everywhere, is to show that what Jesus teaches is the love of God, not to rejoice in the wrath of God. The wrath of God is irrelevant for us.

But it is possible, too, to give a longer answer. In the Old Testament, it is true, illness is sometimes seen as a punishment for sin[7], and this is not explicitly denied in the New Testament. But both testaments make it clear that this has nothing to do with us.

If we are to believe the Psalms, people then as now pointed a finger in judgment at the sick. As an example, Psalm 69(68) shows the psalmist suffering:

> But I am afflicted and in pain;
> let thy salvation, O God, set me on high!

To his suffering is added rejection and humiliation by those around him:

> Thou knowest my reproach,
> and my shame and my dishonour;
> my foes are all known to thee.
> Insults have broken my heart,
> so that I am in despair.
> I looked for pity, but there was none;
> and for comforters, but I found none.
> They gave me poison for food,
> and for my thirst they gave me vinegar to drink.

The psalmist then prays to God that all these ills be visited on them in return:

> Let their own table before them become a snare;
> let their sacrificial feasts be a trap.
> Let their eyes be darkened, so that they cannot see; and make
> their loins tremble continually.

And what is the terrible thing they have done to make them deserve all this?

> Pour out thy indignation upon them,
> and let thy burning anger overtake them . . .
> For they persecute him whom thou hast smitten,
> and him whom thou hast wounded, they afflict still more.

He acknowledges that his affliction comes from God, but it is clearly the duty of those around the sufferer to comfort him. The psalmist expects that God will be outraged at their behaviour and punish them in return. If it is a question of taking sides at all, God expects people to side with the sick.

81

In Psalm 41(40), the psalmist is again sick through his sins:

As for me, I said: "O Lord, be gracious to me;
heal me, for I have sinned against thee!"

Though the psalmist has sinned, God is not his adversary; he can appeal to God confidently for healing. But people are against him:

My enemies say of me in malice:
"When will he die, and his name perish?" . . .
All who hate me whisper together about me;
they imagine the worst for me.

They say: "A deadly thing has fastened upon him;
he will not rise again from where he lies."
Even my bosom friend in whom I trusted,
who ate of my bread, has lifted his heel against me.

The psalmist's neighbours see his illness not as a call for help and compassion, but as an opportunity to accuse and an occasion for satisfaction. They refuse to offer the love which the psalmist knows he can expect from God. In a similar way, when people see or think that Aids is a punishment for sinners or the outpouring of God's wrath, they are accusing those who suffer from it. The disease is seen as a visible sign of guilt and this is somehow thought to license the abandonment of the basic requirements of Christian love—while, in fact, it is an abandonment of the God who is love[8].

The task is to help and comfort

The same theme can be found in the book of Job. One purpose of this book is to challenge the idea that suffering and sickness are God's punishment for sins[9]. Unlike the psalmist, Job does have real friends; they come and sit with him in silence, overcome by the greatness of his suffering[10]. But they try and comfort him in the only way they know, by showing him he is a great sinner and that God is punishing him:

Is it for your fear of him that he reproves you,
and enters into judgment with you?
Is not your wickedness great?
There is no end to your iniquities[11].

Job's friends believe they are taking God's side. But this is not what a suffering man needs to hear; this is no way to comfort:

Miserable comforters are you all . . .
I also could speak as you do,

82

If you were in my place;
I could join words together against you,
and shake my head at you[12].

Once again, people's proper task is to help and comfort the suffering, not to go on about their sins. And so God too in the end is none too pleased with the performance of Job's friends, and has them ask Job to pray for them, so that the way they have spoken may be forgiven them[13].

So there is in one way nothing special about Aids and those who suffer from it, because no diseases and no sufferers can be special. All sufferers are to be helped and comforted in their suffering. Even if we want to say that God punishes, it is the same God who punishes who also demands of us that we act on behalf of those he has punished.

But there is another sense in which people with Aids—who have sometimes been compared to the lepers of biblical times— are indeed special from a Christian point of view. Like the leper, the Aids sufferer is often afflicted with a disease—Kaposi's sarcoma—which progressively disfigures. The comparison is more poignantly apt because Aids sufferers, like lepers, find themselves outcasts. The law of the leper in the Old Testament is stark:

> The leper who has the disease shall wear torn clothes and let the hair of his head hang loose, and he shall cover his lip and cry: "Unclean, unclean." He shall remain unclean as long as he has the disease; he is unclean; he shall dwell alone in a habitation outside the camp[14].

The Old Testament leper may recover; so far, the Aids sufferer cannot. But even before he dies he can, like the leper, be socially dead. He may lose his job and his home, and be shunned by family and friends once the secret gets out. He can end up alone and lonely, cut off from the social mainstream, effectively dwelling in a habitation outside the camp. And this at a time when he most needs support, when he must face up to sickness and his own imminent death. He is like the psalmist who complains:

> My life is spent with sorrow;
> and my years with sighing;
> my strength fails because of my misery,
> and my bones waste away.
>
> I am the scorn of all my adversaries,
> a horror to my neighbours,
> an object of dread to my acquaintances;

those who see me in the street flee from me.
I have passed out of mind like one who is dead;
I have become like a broken vessel[15].

Because we are social animals, this ostracism can be as difficult to bear as the illness that occasions it. In this light, we can appreciate the import of the first healing story in Matthew's gospel:

A leper came to him and knelt before him, saying: "Lord, if you will, you can make me clean." And he stretched out his hand and touched him, saying: "I will; be clean." And immediately his leprosy was cleansed[16].

The leper was ostracised so that others would not be contaminated by contact with him. Jesus is sometimes shown curing people with a word, but not here. He touches this leper. With that simple and fundamental gesture Jesus crosses and abolishes the boundary between ordinary people and the untouchable, drawing the sufferer back into society. For Jesus, there are no dividing walls, nobody is untouchable. The leper is now restored to a fully human life; he can now dwell inside the camp.

Jesus touches the untouchables

Restoration, the abolition of boundaries, touching the untouchable, are constantly stressed in the gospels. Jesus is especially concerned, not only with lepers, but with all those relegated to the margins. According to Matthew, after Jesus cures the leper his next meeting is with a centurion, a member of the Roman occupying forces. Jesus comments that it is those outside, foreigners and strangers, who will inherit the Kingdom, while those who consider themselves the insiders, the "sons of the Kingdom", will find themselves in the outer darkness[17].

Jesus reaches out to the sick and strangers, but above all he seeks out those who have been cast aside for moral reasons, the tax collectors, prostitutes, and others who have seriously broken the law of God:

The Son of man came eating and drinking, and they said: "Behold, a glutton and a drunkard, a friend of tax collectors and sinners!"[18].

Again, Matthew tells us:

As he sat at table in the house, behold, many tax collectors and sinners came and sat down with Jesus and his disciples.

And when the Pharisees saw this, they said to his disciples: "Why does your teacher eat with tax collectors and sinners?"[19].

The question did not come from idle curiosity. The righteous, especially religious teachers, were supposed to stay away from sinners, to have nothing to do with those who by their lives showed themselves to be against God. Jesus completely undermines this approach. For him, the moral outcast is not God's enemy but one who needs healing:

> Those who are well have no need of a physician, but those who are sick. Go and learn what this means: "I desire mercy, and not sacrifice". For I came not to call the righteous, but sinners[20].

For Jesus, God does not lie with the righteous on one side of a divide, while sinners are on the other. Rather, God is to be found where divides are crossed. God's work consists in the restoration of unity, of community. God is for those whom people reject, even when they are rejected for being against God. Jesus offers community to those who have no community except with other outcasts. For this reason, for Jesus, the worst sins are those of division, of judgment, of separation, marking others off, refusing to be one with them.

By judging, we are ourselves judged

In Luke's parable of the Pharisee and the tax collector, the Pharisee thanks God that "he is not like other men, extortioners, unjust, adulterers, or even like this tax collector"[21]. All that the Pharisee says might well be true: many Pharisees were indeed just and upright people. But from Jesus's point of view, the Pharisee's creation of this division, this setting up of sides, is actually working against God. By placing himself on any side at all, the Pharisee places himself on the wrong side. By judging, he is himself judged.

Jesus's view is also central to the Church, his disciples. It is not just one view among others, but the Revelation of God, the mystery in whom and towards whom we are. If Jesus stretches out his hand to bring near those who have been driven off, it is the hand of God that brings them into communion with him. When Jesus dines with tax collectors as well as Pharisees, he shows us the God who makes his sun rise on the evil and on the good and sends rain on the just and the unjust[22]. The Church, made up of those who see the God revealed in Jesus, is not just another group of insiders viewing others as outsiders, one more source of disunity, one more element in the fragmentation of humanity. For St Paul, the Church consists of people who do not come up to the mark, to whom God in Christ has reached out:

> Consider your call, brethren; not many of you were wise according to worldly standards, not many were powerful, not many were of noble birth; but God chose what is foolish in the world to shame the wise, God chose what is weak in the world to shame the strong, God chose what is low and despised in the world, even things that are not, to bring to nothing things that are[23].

The Church is those for whom division has been abolished; it is a sign that there is no divide, a sign of the restoration of unity in Christ, who has broken down the dividing wall of hostility.

The implications of this for the problems raised by Aids are obvious. The mere fact that Aids sufferers often find themselves in the position of outcasts, of untouchables, whether through their own fault or not, makes it especially incumbent on the Church to be a community for them, to be a place where they can turn and be certain of being respected and cared for. That in the West this disease largely, although not exclusively, attacks people whom we or others might think morally suspect is not a reason why we should not concern ourselves with it; it is on the contrary a reason why the Church should be even more concerned to help Aids sufferers than to help those who suffer and die from other, more respectable diseases. While people still condemn each other and continue to erect barriers against sinners, for the Church to be Church, it is essential for us to work to break down those barriers.

---

1 Mt 22.37–40. Here Jesus quotes from Deut 6.4 and Lev 19.18. Cf Mk 12.29–31; Lk 10.25–28.
2 Lk 10.29–37.
3 Mt 25.31–46.
4 Mt 25.34–36, 40.
5 Jn 10.10.
6 See esp. Lev 18.22; 20.13.
7 See e.g. Ps 107(106).17.
8 1 Jn 4.16.
9 Job protests his innocence throughout (see especially ch. 13) We also know from his prologue that he is blameless and upright (1.1), and that God considers him so (1.8).
10 Job 2.11–13.
11 Job 22.4f.

12 Job 16.2,4.
13 Job 42.7–9.
14 Lev 13.45f.
15 Ps 31(30).10–12.
16 Mt 8.2f.
17 Mt 8.5–13.
18 Mt 11.19.
19 Mt 9.10.
20 Mt 9.12.
21 Lk 18.11.
22 Mt 7.24ff.
23 1 Cor 1.26–28.

13 | A call to radical conversion

Bernard Häring CSSR
Catholic moral theologian

I see Aids above all as only one of the symptoms of a gravely sick society: as a challenge to radical conversion, to a whole-person approach to healing, and to a compassionate relationship with the sick and those at risk. All this must, however, be viewed in the larger context of other threats to human health.

Symptom of a sick society

In the not too distant future, Aids may become one of the most serious threats to health in an already unhealthy society. For the time being, however, there are irresponsible ways of behaving which damage more people and ravage human health no less than those that have transmitted the Aids virus. I think, therefore, that we should look at the spread of the particular virus which causes acquired immune deficiency syndrome as a call to foster the spiritual "immunity" which enables us to fight for total spiritual, mental and physical health.

The greatest risk to humanity, and its most humiliating deviation, is the violence and falsehood that have produced the arms race and nuclear deterrence. Only a radical conversion to a non-violent and truthful culture and the most radical "transarmament" for a morally strong "civilian non-violent defence" can save humanity from self-destruction. Many people, after serious reflection, have come to the conclusion that there is no other gateway to a peaceful future and a healthy society than through the "healing power of non-violence"[1]. This implies a changed mentality and lifestyle, which would also enable us to face the problem of Aids.

A second terrible threat to humankind is the poisoning of the entire ecological system. This calls for the same radical new way of thinking, planning and acting.

To make the picture more complete, I mention other factors which at present do greater harm to a larger segment of the population than Aids: uncontrolled cigarette smoking, alcoholism, drug addiction, over-eating, and irresponsible driving. Every year more than 100,000 people are killed and half a million are crippled on our highways around the globe.

Yet we should not minimise the risk that the number of cases of Aids will double at least every year. Already it poisons human relationships, destroys families and innumerable lives.

Medical science has made enormous progress, and many of us benefit from it. And yet we face a massive increase in the number of cases of non-communicable disease, to which is now added Aids—a communicable disease, connected with the most intimate communication. It is a sign of a perverted sexual language, a sexual communication which lacks the truth of faithfulness and responsibility and which has, for many people, become a kind of "sex-consumption" in which the sexual partner is a mere object. Recent research has shown that "sex-tourism" is a main cause of spreading HIV infection, particularly in Africa. Aids is a symptom of a consumer society, of the "non-culture" of having, using, consuming over and against a sexuality of "being" and "being-with-and-for-each-other".

"Do not judge"

Faced with those who suffer from Aids, we should remind ourselves of the warning of Jesus: "Judge not, that you be not judged" (Mt 7.1). We will abstain from a judgmental attitude towards those who are affected by the Aids virus when we realise how deeply Aids is embedded in our sick culture, through our own co-operation in it. Can we really dare to say that we are immune from all those attitudes which spread unhealthiness and increase the risks inherent in unhealthy relationships— a judgmental attitude being one of them? The Aids virus can be spread to thoroughly innocent people by untested blood transfusion or through the sharing of unsterilised needles. A faithful husband or wife can be infected by his or her spouse who was once promiscuous; babies can receive the virus from a blameless mother.

Aids, therefore, cannot be seen in isolation. The words of Jesus in the gospel of Luke (13.3–5) are very much to the point. When people told Jesus of a mass-killing and a disaster, they evidently thought that the victims were worthy of punishment. Jesus warned them, however: "Do you think that these Galileans were worse sinners than all the other Galileans, because they suffered thus? I tell you, No; but unless you repent you will all likewise perish." The fate of those with Aids, both those who acted irresponsibly and those who caught it without any personal fault, is one of the signs of our times calling us to a radical conversion. Societies must become more responsible, and we must all become more responsible persons.

"Be compassionate as your Father is compassionate"

Our response to people with Aids, no matter how they got the infection, is above all one of compassion. Only a sinful self-righteousness ("pseudo-innocence") could prevent us from compassion. We all, as redeemed people, live by divine mercy and compassion. Therefore we owe compassion to each other. Aids is certainly connected with unhealthy human relationships, but in a much broader sense than some might imagine. Only God knows how much some people's compulsive homosexual or heterosexual behaviour may have its roots in their own parents' unhealthy relationships, or those of other people or communities. If we have somehow understood the whole complex problem of Aids we can surely, even on the basis of a humanist ethics, understand that our proper response should be to promote and to cultivate healthy human relationships throughout society: genuine, faithful love, compassion and loving care, respect and mutual understanding, patient dialogue. There are inner resources to be awakened by healthy and healing relationships, resources which offer a kind of immunity against the dark powers, against our selfish selves. Giving others an advance of trust helps them to forgive themselves and to find a new, healthy trust in their own inner resources.

The lepers in the Hebrew culture of the time of Jesus, and even today in some cultures, were treated as outcasts and harshly despised as sinners punished by God. Such rejection cannot happen to people with Aids, at least never by those who call themselves Christians. By treating them as outcasts we would degrade ourselves and our communities. We ourselves become spiritually and psychologically healthier if we meet the sick in full respect and offer, where needed, compassionate help and care without the slightest judgmental attitude.

An ethics of responsibility

The horrifying system of mutual deterrence, the ecological crisis, the deterioration of human health through various forms of addiction and irresponsible lifestyles, and now the crisis of Aids, require us to become responsible persons, form responsible communities and societies, and concentrate on education for responsibility. Yet it is not possible to sharpen people's consciences for responsibility on this one point, Aids, unless we educate ourselves and help others to develop an overall sense of responsibility for our own health, for the health of others, for healthy human relationships, and for peace and justice.

Past and present experience proclaim loudly that a rigid and one-sided emphasis on sexual morality is counter-productive and causes dangerous reactions. Sexual morality is of paramount importance, but education for sexual responsibility can operate only if people understand deeply their responsibility for their own well-being.

Modern people reject taboos and they reject moral norms almost as strongly, especially in the field of sexual relationships, if the norms smack of authoritarian imposition. Norms and prohibitions work in the long run only if the scale of values on which they are grounded is communicated in a convincing and attractive manner.

Today's moral theology, based on a long tradition, gives great weight to teleological argument. That means asking what kind of norms serve human dignity, human well-being, and express human responsibility and co-responsibility best in view of the highest and most urgent human values.

In the effort to educate for responsibility in all fields of human life, interpersonal and social, we must allow people to argue, to ask critical questions, even to express their dissent frankly if they find the norms unconvincing. Only through a deep insight into human values can we help each other to find strong and effective motivations.

90

Integrated sexual education

Only after all this do I dare to offer frankly some reflections on sexual education. What is to be said can be understood within the individual's fundamental option to be and to become, and to act ever more as a responsible person. Sexuality has to do with reciprocity, with being-with, with deep human relationships. Only the loving, respectful and faithful person can be a sexually responsible person. An encounter between people of the same or different sex is communication. The sexual encounter is language: either truthful or deceptive. In casual sexual-genital activity, the user tries to speak the language of love while lying to himself or herself, and to the other. He uses language of belonging and of fidelity without having any such thing in mind. Prostitution and promiscuity are in themselves irresponsible: they are false, deceptive communication with all the resulting frustrations and degradations. Those who have not learned to bring their sexual drives under control run the immediate danger of becoming compulsive users, consumers, in the field of sexual activity.

I once asked a compulsive homosexual whether fear of Aids might not help him to resist. It could not. He would need a total re-orientation, a radical conversion, religiously speaking, and great endurance in a process of total healing. Similarly, others cannot overcome the smoking habit, gravely damaging their own health and the health of others, unless they find a strong motivation to become free and act freely for a genuine love of self and others.

We cannot postpone educating for responsibility in view of Aids until we have educated people for a general responsibility. But in the urgent task of pointing out some of the most evident motives and norms for sexual responsibility in order to face the situation caused by Aids we must never forget the broader task of helping each other to act as responsible persons in all of our life and to see the call for chastity as a call to genuine love and responsibility.

Sex and Aids

In some parts of the world more than 70 per cent of homosexuals who have frequently changed their partners are already infected by the HIV virus. Yet many studies on the spread of Aids in Africa have given more than sufficient evidence that heterosexual promiscuity and prostitution are the main causes of the rapid spread of this disease.

In several major cities of Africa, including tourist centres like Nairobi and Kinshasa, a high percentage of prostitutes are already infected by Aids, while it is likely that only very few of the prostitutes were carriers ten years ago. Disastrous social conditions in new urban centres, the lack of roots, and often bitter hunger, drive young girls and women to prostitution. After visits to prostitutes, many men have contaminated their wives, and these women infect their babies either in the womb or by breast-feeding: "Two thirds of infants born to infected mothers are infected, and half of infected infants develop Aids within two years".[2]

Numerous publications also offer the shocking insight that "sex-tourism", organised by western profiteers, provides African or Filipino girls for visitors, which further spreads the HIV virus around the globe. From the moral point of view we can only sharply denounce the business which degrades the women of the poorer countries.

There will be further heart-breaking moral questions raised by Aids. In families where one of the spouses knows he or she is infected, he must do his very best to avoid infection of his spouse. We can fully understand that doctors and political leaders are urging men to use condoms to prevent infection. But it must also be repeated that even this may not be fully safe. However, from the viewpoint of traditional moral theology we may refer in this regard to the "minus malum", by which the lesser evil should be tolerated rather than condemned, to avoid a forseeable greater evil.

In the light of Aids, old burning issues of moral theology turn up with new ardour. In many parts of the Catholic world, divorced or abandoned spouses who have had several sexual partners during the year have received easy absolution in their Easter confession, while divorced and remarried Catholics who live a faithful and stable civil marriage were refused absolution unless they promised to abstain from sexual intercourse. Sometimes the wife kept this promise, while her husband turned to prostitutes or other persons. What should be our approach to this problem now? Should we not heed the appeal of the great majority of bishops at the Synod on the Family in Rome (1980) to study whether the Roman Church might not learn something from the Eastern Orthodox Churches, which use the age-old practice of healing compassion (oikonomia) with divorced people whose first marriage is hopelessly dead?

If we want our teaching on sexual morality to motivate and move people from within, we can no longer allow ourselves to proclaim that all sins against chastity are mortal sins; we cannot express condemnation of "abortion, sterilisation and contraception" without using even a semi-colon to separate things so different in their gravity.

Aids requires the Churches to fight against promiscuity and prostitution as well as against adultery. Revelation and human insight offer enough convincing reasons to condemn these aberrations which now, additionally, have become the main vehicles of Aids. But if we focus on sentences such as "each conjugal act must be open for procreation" or put the sexual intercourse of firmly promised fiancés (out of human weakness or an "erroneous conscience") on the same level as promiscuity and/or prostitution then we should not be surprised if we do not get a hearing from modern people. It is a matter of wise perspectives and convincing emphasis. The facts about the transmission of Aids and other reasons should persuade us to concentrate more convincingly on major evils and dangers. If at the same time we stress the overall need for education for responsibility and discernment, people will also be more attentive to those norms that are less urgent. In this regard we can surely learn constantly from the preaching of Jesus and of the Apostles.

1 Bernard Häring, *The Healing Power of Peace and Non-Violence* (St Paul Publications, Slough, 1986).
2 *AIFO*, January 1987, p. 17.

PART V | Pastoral approaches

14 | Aids and sex education

Justin Price OSB
Director of health education at Ampleforth College

A short time ago I wrote, "Anyone planning an educational programme to contain the spread of Aids is involved in a running battle which he cannot afford to lose. We have to keep abreast, and preferably ahead, of an enemy whose characteristics, present disposition and likely future movements are uncertain but increasingly menacing on an ever-widening front." (*The Tablet*, 14 February, 1987). Such anthropomorphic language is vivid but misleading. It creates the illusion that responsibility for the outcome of the current threat to the heterosexual population can be shifted onto someone or something else: homosexuals, the promiscuous, the KGB, the CIA, God. All have been blamed at one time or another. I intended the metaphor to refer to the Aids virus, even though it appears to attribute to it a malevolent intelligence it does not possess.

In fact, the virus itself is a fragile and all but impotent parasite, completely dependent for its survival and transmission on its human host. It is people, predominantly through their sexual activity, whose present way of living has made the Aids virus so widespread a danger. In the absence of any vaccine or cure, all hope of victory in the battle against Aids rests on our success in learning to control and direct our own sexual drives into safe channels. The battle is likely to be a long one, and the real enemy is within us, betrayed by confusion of thought and feeling, truncated vision, and weakness of will in sexual matters.

The aim of educators must be to bring first themselves, then the young, to reflect and act on these matters. The teacher's job is to devise a strategy which stirs up the fundamental questions raised by Aids in the minds of the young and leads them to change their attitudes and behaviour. The virus is not yet widespread in the heterosexual population and there is little current danger to the majority of sexually active young people, but they are without doubt a very vulnerable group.

Wherever possible, the Christian teacher will want to influence his or her students towards chastity, not just because it gives the maximum degree of protection against Aids, but for all the right and good reasons that have always been true. It may

97

be that the threat of Aids will predispose youngsters to listen and adopt a chaste lifestyle when in the past they might have shrugged off such arguments without much thought. It may also be that this is a particular time of grace, enabling people to make changes in their lives which might once have been too much for them. The teacher needs to be sensitive to all this, and not jump too readily to the conclusion that the call to chastity will meet with no response.

Encouraging a climate of respect

How might a teacher approach a class of 16-year-old boys and girls in a Catholic school? Whenever possible, education about Aids should form part of a broader programme of health and sex education. Like all aspects of education for personal relationships, it needs an open and trusting atmosphere, more especially since at this stage of the Aids campaign the teacher's primary role is to help young people reflect and decide on the changes in their lifestyle made necessary by Aids. To do this, the teacher must create in his or her class a climate of genuineness and respect, which are encouraged when the teacher's main concern is to listen carefully to what the students have to say about themselves. In the end, the only moral judgment which is fully effective is that of individual conscience. The teacher's influence will ultimately be greater if he listens more readily than he speaks.

It is a delicate matter for a teacher to ask a group to talk personally about sexual matters without seeming intrusive or even voyeuristic. He or she might offer them the protection of working in small, self-selected groups within the class, taking care to negotiate with them the terms of confidentiality which will bind them all before they start to discuss sensitive topics.

The teacher does not want them to talk about the virus or Aids as such, but about the way in which their sexual attitudes and practices could maintain it and spread it. He wants to bring them to a point where they can accept full responsibility for their share in the problem, and can if necessary radically reassess their attitudes and change any which may be dangerous to moral, physical, or spiritual health.

The approach suggested here is based on the well-tried approach to counselling developed by Dr Gerard Egan[1]. The strategy has, in broad terms, three stages. In the first, the teacher's aim is to help the pupils develop a coherent and honest picture of their own current sexual attitudes, expectations, experiences and behaviour. The goal of the second stage is to get them to see how this picture changes in the light, or shadow, of the Aids threat, and then to consider what changes they might make in their lives in response. The third stage is to help them choose, implement and maintain those changes which are likely to be effective.

The first stage: current attitudes and behaviour

One way of exploring the current attitudes and experience of young people is to encourage discussion of a few rather personal questions in small groups. "How many sexual partners do you think people like you might have over the next five years?" "Would you take the Church's teaching on sex before marriage as a personal ideal?" "In what kind of relationships and circumstances do you think people like you might have some experience of sex with another person?" In this way, their attention is focussed from the beginning on their own involvement, though there is no attempt as yet to get them to shift their own perspective, simply to describe their own position to themselves as clearly as possible and to report on it in general terms to the whole class.

When they report back, the picture which all too frequently emerges is that most of the boys expect to have ten or more sexual partners over the next five years. They will know some of their partners well; others will be "one night stands". Girls in the class are usually more restrained in their predictions, but only a very few among either sex say that they accept and try to live by the Christian ideal of premarital chastity.

Even allowing for the bragging factor—although the class will openly scoff at any group which makes too extravagant a claim for the predicted number of partners—these findings are likely to run contrary to what the teacher would like to hear. It is important that the teacher's reaction should be to check that he or she has understood clearly what they are saying and get them to complete and clarify the picture as far as is possible in the circumstances of the classroom.

The second stage: impact of Aids

It would be tempting, but a mistake, for the teacher to pass immediately from these revelations to an attempt to persuade them of the necessity and advantages of premarital chastity. Instead, the teacher should explore with them the likely consequences of the imminent appearance of Aids among

99

sexually active young people. The need for a wide range of changes in social and sexual behaviour will soon become apparent. This leads them to see that they form one of the front line groups and their sense of responsibility for the future is awakened.

Without doubt, the new element in their awareness is that of fear. They are, rightly, worried—often very worried. There is no need to inflate that fear by playing up the dangers. On the contrary, it is wise to reassure those who are heterosexually active that they are unlikely to have contracted the virus, and are unlikely to do so next weekend. Most of them have time to change their sexual expectations or behaviour before the virus comes knocking at their door.

It is true that some 16-year-olds may be immediately at risk. They may have travelled to countries where the virus is well-established among the heterosexual population or lurking in the local blood banks. Some may be homosexually active or taking drugs intravenously. They could themselves also be a source of infection for others, even for the group sitting there in front of the teacher. Individual counselling should be made available to any child who believes he or she may be at risk.

Moment of decision

For most pupils, the anxiety generated by their perception of the spread of Aids will be enough to make them want to change their behaviour. But before they are ready to face the hard option of chastity, they will want to explore all the alternatives. They will want to know about safer forms of sexual behaviour and in particular about the use of the condom as a protective.

The government campaign advocates its use but avoids discussion of the condom's limitations. In supplying the full facts, it is important to stay within the "real life" context of the pupils, so that they may judge how effective a condom is likely to be for people like them in circumstances like theirs. Once all the other preventive measures have been explored the effectiveness of premarital chastity and fidelity to one partner in marriage becomes self-evidently the safest, if not the easiest practical option. No further medical argument is needed.

The pupils are then presented with a moment of decision, as they weigh the residual risk of intercourse with a condom and its possible consequences for themselves and others against the cost to themselves of adopting the harder option of premarital chastity.

100

The choice at this point of premarital abstention from intercourse on medical grounds does not, of course, amount to an acceptance of Christian chastity as such. But set alongside their newly-realised sense of responsibility for the future, it may make them think again about the over-valuation of the genital expression of sexuality that they have received from society. They may be ready for the first time to question the foundations of their behaviour and to look for something better as well as safer. For after the realisation that they must change their sexual behaviour or risk death may follow the acknowledgment that their sexual expectations were not, as they had assumed, liberating and life-enhancing, but potentially deeply destructive of individual persons and societies.

At this moment, confronting the menace of Aids and the medical logic of chastity, the pupils may feel caught between two great fears: the fear that death will be insinuated into their lives through unguarded sexual intercourse, and the fear of a bland and lonely life without it. The poverty of our culture, in which all expression of affection seems to have been smothered by or subsumed into the genital, comes suddenly into stark relief. They see the diminution of the heart implied in the belief that sexual love alone can satisfy our deepest longings. The escape from this double trap lies in the exploration of friendship and the rediscovery of God.

The teacher should be ready for this transition from the negative to the positive, from the fear of death and disease to questioning of the significance of sexual feelings. When it occurs, he or she may be able to help young people articulate their need for divine as well as human intimacy and so see this quest for the ultimately satisfying relationship in the perspective of faith. In the long-term, the role of the teacher, beyond the scope of this chapter, is crucially important in the pastoral care of young people and the renewal of our understanding of chastity.

The third stage: the practice of chastity

Learning to live chastely involves more than the simple desire or decision to do so. The call to complete premarital chastity presents a tremendous challenge to young people who are already sexually active. Because of the strength of the feelings and habits involved, it is unlikely that most of them will be able to change their lives in one great leap. There is bound to be a struggle, with times of success and times of failure. It seems to

101

me that the teacher and others involved in the continuing pastoral care of young people have a double task. They must both encourage them in persevering towards chastity and at the same time acknowledge the possibility of failure in self-control or conviction, and prepare them for the consequences that could follow.

Sometimes, the teacher or pastor will meet an out-and-out self-centred hedonist, who is apparently unmoved by discussion, reflection, or any sense of responsibility to the future. The teacher needs to believe that the same advice he or she has offered to all the pupils may nevertheless open a small crack in the hedonistic facade which may be the beginning of a movement towards a higher kind of love.

The content of lessons or discussion on Aids in a Christian school will therefore include all the relevant medical and preventive information, but must set it in the context of God's care for his people and our co-responsibility with him as stewards of creation. The Christian teacher must count on God's grace working in the lives of young people at risk.

It should go without saying that the way of life of the teacher must be in line with his or her own commitment to Christian chastity. Young people talking to their teachers about sexual matters must know exactly where they, and the Church, stand; and must sense that it has brought them to a happy integration in their own lives.

In the long-term

What of the longer term? We may assume that, at best, any educational campaign will succeed only in managing rather than annihilating the spread of Aids. This means that teachers and parents, looking at their classes and families now, must fear that some of them may die in spite of every educational and preventive measure.

Preparing people to cope with the personal consequences of Aids in the family, in the circle of friends, and in the community of parish or school, is an important part of the long-term educational response to the crisis. We must prepare ourselves and our students for grief, for the search for meaning in the midst of affliction; we must be ready to face in ourselves and in others the inevitable questions about the loving nature of a God who can permit such a thing to strike those whom his Son loves so much. The depth of faith required to ride such a storm of questioning and despair can only be a gift for which we must pray.

There are many underlying causes of the promiscuity which has enabled Aids to spread. Without undervaluing personal responsibility, we can accept that the fragility of the family and the pernicious commercial use of sex have played a part. The current generation of adolescent youth is so much at risk because attitudes to sexual activity and self-control have been deeply conditioned by the way in which the sexual drive has been manipulated in our culture. Advertising, popular music, teen magazines, videos, soft and hard pornography are all at work to detach sexual activity from love, marriage and the family and set it spinning free in the teenage subculture. As part of a long-term educational strategy, we need to teach young people to take a close and careful look at this conditioning process, in the hope that through reflection they will be able to disentangle themselves from it to some extent.

We must also give them something to put in its place. The Church must make explicit a positive and inspiring theology of sex if its response to Aids is not to appear a mere relapse into the fears and prohibitions of the past. We must change our perspective on human sexuality and give real assent to it as a sacramental participation in the love of God, of which chastity is both a recognition and a celebration.

1. Gerard Egan, *The Skilled Helper* (Brooks/Cole Publishing, 3rd edition 1986).

15 | Education in the Christian community

Anthony Clark

Continuing education officer for Westminster Diocese Education Service

The focus of this article is the process of education of the Catholic community—the homes, parishes, schools, clergy and leadership of the Church in Britain—to come to terms in a positive and Christian manner with Aids, a disease that is recent, deadly and connected with the most important of human processes, that of sexuality and reproduction. The aim of the education process is to help Catholics to become informed about the disease, to find ways to interpret it in a Christian way, and to approach people with Aids in a manner that is not dominated by fear, but rather by a desire to help.

However, before one can even begin to look at the process of education in the community, something should be said on what is often called "the loss of innocence" but which might be more accurately described as the loss of reticence. Even those who grew up during the '60s find the overtness and explicitness of current information and discussion on sexual matters more than they were ever accustomed to.

Many parents, for example, have the feeling that their children are being exposed to knowledge that should rather wait until they are a little older. On a personal note, my own five-year-old child has asked me if I ever use a condom or have Aids. With regret, we must simply accept that the threat of Aids means that clear and explicit knowledge and open discussion form the best basis for safety and protection for the individual, the family and the community.

The basic issues

The issues raised by Aids are not in the first place theological or moral, rather the practical issues which are to be informed by a Christian approach and understanding. They include the following: How to protect oneself and one's family from contracting Aids; how far to co-operate with the public programmes of education and prevention; whether to find out if one is a carrier or not; whether to marry or have children if one is; whether to inform others, and which others.

The issues it raises for society include: how much money to devote to research, care and education; who should be tested and how HIV-carriers and people with Aids should be cared for; and what precautions should be taken in public places such as hospitals and schools.

Specifically, the Catholic community must decide how to respond positively within parishes and schools to meet the needs of the Aids patient and HIV-carrier; and how to encourage positive attitudes, listen and educate in the face of fear and prejudice.

Many of the decisions to be made in the community depend on us having firm information about the disease. This information is not finally available and thus our decisions are made under conditions of uncertainty, and our policies based on caution. Policies and practices must be developed which assume that one's neighbour may be a carrier, which do not entail great changes in daily life but do require a major change in current sexual behaviour.

Sources of attitudes

A major influence on attitudes has been the tabloid press which in particular has raised subconscious memories and fears connected with plagues. In this atmosphere self-protection and survival instincts, notorious for being short-sighted and blind to the common good, come to the fore. Furthermore, the press has exaggerated the degree to which Aids is connected with homosexuality. While most cases of Aids in the West have so far occurred among homosexuals, the issues are separate from those raised by homosexuality and must be kept distinct. The response of the community must be an education programme which goes beyond primitive instincts or stereo-typed attitudes.

Christian attitudes reflect those of Christ, whose ministry and preaching were characterised by forgiveness, healing and concern for outcasts. All these characteristics should be evident and real on the part of our communities.

Insofar as Aids is contracted through moral fault, Christians should forgive individuals. There can be no atmosphere of "approving" the disease as a punishment. Equally, Christians must avoid imputing moral guilt to Aids sufferers, some of whom are haemophiliacs, faithful spouses, babies, and so on.

Both at the level of supporting medical research programmes which seek a cure, at the level of prayer and laying on of hands, and at the level of counselling, Christians should be at the forefront of efforts to heal all the sick, including those with Aids.

Christian communities should make every effort to find ways of showing that Aids patients and carriers are not outcasts in any way. Aids challenges parishes and schools to examine the degree to which they already treat the sick and outcasts (including the poor, handicapped, and racial minorities) and to review their attitudes towards them. The very real and deep challenge to everyone must not be underestimated, however. We are all very susceptible to irrational fear and cannot simply affirm that we would not ever reject an Aids sufferer until we have worked through the possibility that we might contract the disease ourselves and put ourselves and our families at risk because of our Christian concern.

Cardinal Hume in his article in *The Times* of 7 January wrote:

A radical change in popular attitudes is possible, indeed necessary. Many in recent years have become convinced of the need to embrace a simpler, healthier lifestyle in order to enjoy a fuller, longer life. We are already changing deep-rooted habits in eating, drinking, smoking and exercise. How much greater is the necessity to rediscover the joy of faithful love and lasting marriage. It calls for self-discipline, restraint and a new awareness. Such a profound change in society also needs a comprehensive campaign of public education and persuasion.

This quote indicates the importance of reinforcing the Christian message of the dignity of every human and the positive Christian approach to sexuality, motivated by true human happiness rather than the fear of threat to health and life. It is especially important to emphasise that individuals who are homosexually oriented can achieve happiness and humanity in their lives without physical sexual expression.

Christians must also react to media and advertising messages with discernment. The contradictions within the media are well-exemplified by the juxtaposition in tube stations of the Aids poster put out by the Department of Health and Social Security with a Club 18-30 advertisement for holidays "You wouldn't dare tell Father about". Christians need to become critically aware of the influence of the media and learn to evaluate the processes involved.

Despite the clear priorities for education about Aids, there remains the very real question of how to promote the educational process. There are no simple or quick techniques for achieving changes in moral awareness and behaviour. At one level the process is the same as that used to educate people, for example, to the dangers of smoking. But at a deeper level it is part of the struggle to respond to the challenge of the Gospel. In the parable of the sower, the message is received in a variety of ways and people grow in their understanding. Conversion to the teaching of the Gospel is a lifelong process which is never fully achieved.

Education of the clergy

At a diocesan level in particular there is a need for a sustained and thorough education programme for the clergy. They are at the forefront of efforts to form Christian attitudes in the community and may be a resource for individuals and families touched in any way by the disease. A study programme for the clergy on Aids might include the following:

a. A thorough presentation of the medical facts;
b. A study of the implications of the disease for marriage preparation and marriage counselling;
c. Understanding of the ethos and thought patterns of young people;
d. A full discussion of the ethical implications;
e. An introduction to appropriate counselling approaches and advice on where to get further training;
f. A full study of prudent precautions to be followed in parish and liturgical activities.

Listening to the insights of workers and counsellors who are already involved with people with Aids can be very useful in setting out agendas and points in this training programme, which should ideally be led by the bishop in conjunction with medical, educational, theological and counselling advisers. Such study days for the clergy have already begun in several dioceses.

Clergy will increasingly have to face dilemmas which are not yet resolvable. In marriage preparation, should a priest advise a worried young couple to seek tests to discover if either is HIV-positive? How might a priest cope if one party is found

107

positive and the couple are forced to reconsider their planned marriage? Does he have the counselling skills and confidence to help the couple? If there are reasonable grounds for suspecting that a person may be HIV-positive, should a marriage proceed without a test? Is concealment of the fact that one is a carrier or at high risk of being a carrier grounds for subsequent annulment? Yet the very process of advising a test must be carefully considered, not least for financial reasons, as a positive test may have major implications for mortgage and insurance arrangements. A priest needs to be aware of the consequences of any advice he gives.

Further, priests need to be aware of the skills required to respond to the families of Aids sufferers. In some cases the news of their son's illness is also the first intimation to parents that he is homosexual. Deep shock and strong emotions, possibly very hostile, are the common initial reactions of such parents, which may be followed by the yearning that their child might rather die of a "respectable" disease.

There is evidence that the Aids epidemic has caused a reemergence of open harassment and discrimination against homosexuals. The letter on the Pastoral Care of Homosexuals issued by the Congregation for the Doctrine of the Faith in October 1986 includes a timely reminder of the priest's duty to speak out against such prejudice:

> It is deplorable that homosexual persons have been and are the object of violent malice in speech or action. Such treatment deserves condemnation from pastors whenever it occurs.

Towards a deeper understanding

The best learning often occurs in response to a specific challenge, whether it is something that is being highlighted by the press— "Will Princess Diana wear gloves or not when she shakes hands with an Aids patient"—or something that has come up locally—"Ambulance driver refuses kiss of life to accident patient for fear of Aids."

Christians are looked to for arguments and witness for the positions we hold, and there is a real thirst on the part of many to do this confidently and effectively. Perhaps the most important aspect of any education programme for individuals on a subject such as Aids is that of learning "moral literacy", the ability to think and analyse for oneself. This process is called "formation of conscience" and includes the following:

a. finding out the facts;
b. prayer;
c. studying and listening to the traditions and teaching of the Church;
d. reading the Scriptures;
e. seeking out the advice of the wise and informed in the community.

As, increasingly, Catholics are encouraged to make autonomous moral decisions, they are moving towards a deeper understanding of the reasons for Church teaching on various topics and away from a blind acceptance of authoritative positions.

An education programme for adults should also clarify the distinction that must be made between the stating of moral positions and the appropriate pastoral response to individuals. There remains for many Catholics a real tension in this distinction, which, however, follows the example of Christ. In the story in St John's gospel of the woman taken in adultery, Christ intervenes in the attempt to stone her to death but sends her away with the commandment to sin no more. Christians are called to hold on to the teaching of ideals, such as no adultery or divorce, and at the same time make a positive response to adulterers and divorcees. This tension is particularly sharp as the Church asserts that homosexual acts are immoral but at the same time insists that we must respond positively to homosexuals in a caring and loving way.

Community expectations used to be very powerful in determining acceptable behaviour and attitudes. However, since the turn of the century they have been declining in their power, culminating with the "I'll do what I like" mentality of a number of people in the '70s. There can be no return to the tighter social control hankered after by some, but there can be a strengthening of community expectations so that young people especially are encouraged to behave more responsibly for their own sake and the community's sake. One good way of achieving this is through the exchange and discussion of views between individuals in the context of small groups.

Aids and the chalice

It needs to be made absolutely clear that no change in current practices in Christian churches is called for in the light of the threat of Aids. Aids cannot be passed on through the possible tiny amounts of saliva that might remain on the lip of the chalice. The virus is, in any event, destroyed by alcohol and Aids patients will themselves avoid receiving the chalice as they are threatened by all the common infections that it just might carry which are no threat to ordinary people but which are potentially lethal to them.

For many people used to a more traditional approach to education, the more open approach is not easy. The best learning occurs through shared information, and discussion of experience and expectations. The Christian response to moral issues should be to learn to say "no" from inner conviction and to say "yes" out of concern for those in need. This is begun by addressing three fears: the fear of the disease, the fear of sexuality and the fear of death. This is achieved by a deeper response to the challenge of Christ in the gospels, the challenge to grow in love.

The Catholic school and Aids

To complete this article, I would like to add a few words about the specific policies which may be required within Catholic schools.

The primary responsibility of the school governors is to ensure that Christian attitudes are embodied concretely in the structures and policies of the school. Since the 1986 Education Act, this includes the overview of the sex education programme being followed in the school. During their 1987 Low Week meeting the Bishops' Conference of England and Wales also recommended that there be a review of sex education guidelines in the light of Aids.

The single most important contribution governors can make is to help in the education of parents. Together with the head and staff they could run evening meetings for parents to allow them to voice their fears and come to terms with the threat of Aids through informed discussion.

Heads' responsibilities

Guidelines were circulated to schools in 1986 by the Department of Education and Science advising heads that they should ensure in a non-alarming way that certain types of behaviour are simply not tolerated. These included: no biting; no games involving blood; no tattooing; no sharing of razors or

110

toothbrushes; no classroom experiments involving a pupil's own blood.

There is no evidence of the virus being passed on through saliva and it is creating a false threat to suggest that it might be. The guidelines do emphasise, however, that there is no danger from shared eating utensils, shared musical instruments, etc.

The parents of a child who is HIV-positive are not legally required to inform the school. They are advised to think very carefully about whom they inform and if there is any doubt about the maintenance of confidentiality, then they should not pass on the information.

If the head teacher does know that a child in the school is a carrier then there must be clear policies worked out with the governors which include the need to maintain confidentiality so that the pupils and parents do not know who the child is. Some problems will be avoided if this policy of confidentiality is made known to parents before there is a case in the school. At the same time there must be a clear "need to know" hierarchy which will probably include only a senior teacher and the school nurse.

Current medical advice is to treat spills and "accidents" involving bodily fluids as "biohazards", not only because of Aids but because of the possible presence of other viruses such as Hepatitis B. Splashes of blood and other accidents only need mopping up with alcohol wipes, dilute bleach, or, on carpeted areas, a combination of disinfectant and detergent, to be completely safe. However, given the evidence that in the rough and tumble of ordinary family life an Aids sufferer does not pass on the virus to any other member of his or her family, excessive concern in these areas is not called for.

Borough education and medical officers may but need not necessarily be informed unless the child is a haemophiliac. They should also be given details of the set policy of the school in the case of an Aids carrier being known in the school.

It must be emphasised how critical confidentiality is. A child can easily through ignorance and prejudice be hounded from a school although their presence presents no threat or danger at all. At the same time it must be hoped that parents and others will become sufficiently aware not to respond in this negative and fearful fashion.

16 Aids in Ireland

Brian Power
Member of the Dublin Diocesan Task Force on Aids

It was during 1986 that most Irish people became gradually aware of the existence of Aids as a threat to human well-being in their own country as well as abroad. By the end of that year, nine deaths from Aids were known to have occurred in Ireland. Statistics from the microbiology department of University College, Dublin, showed that at that time 502 people had tested HIV-positive. Those most affected were haemophiliacs, to whom it was believed there was no further risk, and intravenous drug abusers, among whom it was feared that the virus would spread rapidly.

The incursion of Aids into Irish society differed from that in the United States and England, but is similar to that in Scotland, because a much higher proportion of those affected have been drug abusers sharing needles rather than homosexual or bisexual men. This may have been due in part to the work of Gay Health Action, who, as early as May 1985, had begun to distribute information about Aids and in October of that year established a support group for those infected with the virus.

Task force formed

I am a Catholic priest engaged in parish work who, through my background in social research, became involved in the study and prevention of drug abuse at local level. Early in 1986 the Dun Laoghaire Drugs Awareness Group, of which I was a member, learned that several young people we knew had been infected with HIV. As a result, we felt obliged to inform ourselves about its nature and effects.

In October 1986, the director of the drugs awareness programme in the archdiocese of Dublin, Fr Paul Lavelle, set up a Task Force on Aids, chaired by Dr Geoffrey Dean, which I was invited to join. The task force's report was completed in February 1987, shortly after the Irish hierarchy issued their statement on Aids.

The bishops emphasised the need for a response to the emerging crisis on two levels. Firstly, it required "a compassionate and caring attitude towards those who are its victims". The role of the Christian community as a sign of

112

Christ's love, especially for the marginalised and the suffering, was strongly asserted. At the second level, that of prevention of the further spread of the disease, the bishops said that it "would be sad if the response to this major threat were to be reduced simply to a debate about free needles or easy availability of condoms". The real issues of drug abuse and sex would have to be confronted. Greater support for education on the use of drugs and on "the precious gift of sexual love" were needed.

"The only reliable safeguard against contracting the virus by sexual means", the bishops stressed, "is through faithfulness to one's partner in marriage and through self-denial and self-restraint outside of marriage. It is vital that this be made crystal clear."

When the House of Bishops of the Church of Ireland issued a Lenten statement on Aids on 13 March 1987, it was more strongly worded than that of the Catholic hierarchy. It pointed out that while some of those who are infected with HIV acquired it passively, "by far the larger group of those infected received the virus in an 'active' manner, especially through homosexual activity and drug abuse". The need for a Christian response of prayer and compassion was given due precedence, for "each sufferer is a person whom God loves and to whom we must also show his love". On the other hand, "we must also refute those false prophets who have misled people into believing that there is no moral limit to human freedom". The statement recognised that governments have an obligation "to do everything possible to make people aware of the dangers of Aids and to provide advice as to how it may be contained". It concluded, however, with the caution that "only by a reawakening to the value of self-discipline, restraint, fidelity, and awareness of the consequences of a failure to abide by such principles will disaster be averted".

Education and care

In its report, submitted on 10 February 1987, the task force stated that its members were in general agreement that "the main areas in which the Church could respond were education and care". They agreed on the need for an open telephone line, linked to an information centre staffed by professionals, which would provide accurate information and act as a referral agency to appropriate services. Liaison with the Department of Health, the task force realised, would be essential in order to establish such a service.

Various other proposals were made, including the suggestion that the Church might sponsor a counselling service for people with Aids who requested it. Key members of the task force planned to continue to liaise with the Department of Health. The report also admitted that "the care of Aids victims and HIV-positive persons and their families in the home, hospital and hospice settings needs a great deal of further thought and attention".

So far, the principal results of the task force's deliberations have been programmes to educate the clergy and the formation of parish groups. The diocesan task force's work has not ended, however. At a press conference in Maynooth on 11 March 1987, the Irish bishops announced that they would establish a national task force with a pastoral care coordinator, Fr Paul Lavelle, to combat Aids at the levels of care for those infected and education for prevention.

The Christian Churches must accept that they will have an important role in forming attitudes of compassion towards people suffering from and because of Aids, and in dispelling ignorance and myths about the nature and transmittability of the virus. In Ireland, too, religious congregations engaged in working with the sick could exercise a considerable impact on the provision of services and on the way that society responds to the needs of people with Aids and their families.

A great deal of planning will have to be devoted to the provision of care and counselling facilities and it must be admitted that very little headway appeared to have been made at the time of writing. It is in this area that we may hope to learn the most from the experience of those in Britain and the United States.

17 | The invitation to meet Christ

Timothy Radcliffe OP
Prior of Blackfriars, Oxford

"The Catholic Church and Aids" was the title of a conference held at Spode Centre, Staffordshire, in early November 1986. Over a hundred nurses and doctors, priests and religious, social workers, counsellors and concerned Catholics met to try and work out a practical strategy for the Church in this country to serve people with Aids. Several conferences have been held since then and more are planned; I wish, therefore, in this chapter, to present some of the insights and proposals that emerged that weekend because I believe they remain valid.

People with Aids are terminally ill. What we must offer them is, in essence, just what we already offer to those who are sick and dying. There is nothing inherently special about Aids except our reaction to it. If conferences need to be held on the Church and Aids and this book must be written, it is because we are forced to fight hard to hold on to this fundamental insight in the face of the hysteria that the illness generates in some people.

The flight from chaos

It has always been the Church's duty to fight superstition and mythology. All sorts of illnesses have in the past been perceived as signs of God's wrath against sin, including cancer, smallpox and leprosy. But in the clear light of the Gospel we can see that we are simply being faced with people who are ill and dying. So the first thing that the Church can offer is a sense of the ordinariness of people with Aids, and that is why the real victory must be won at parish level. We are challenged to ensure that Aids patients are visited, prayed for and taken communion, like other sick people. The most serious question that the Aids crisis raises for the Church is this: how effective is our ministry for all the sick people in our parishes. Do we remember them?

If the basis of any pastoral care for people with Aids is that they simply be seen as they are and not mythologised into bearers of chaos and disorder, then we must begin with education, which alone can set us free from hysteria.

115

It is worth reflecting for a moment, however, on the purpose and goal of our educational programmes, otherwise they may fail to liberate us into effective pastoral action. It is, obviously, a priority to educate both children and adults about the nature of the virus and its means of transmission. Only this solid understanding will give people the confidence to work with those who have Aids, and only this information will slow the spread of the virus. But all the Churches have insisted that it is not enough to teach people about safer sex, that we have the authority and obligation to assert the moral dimension. This is true, but we may then ask ourselves what is the purpose of moral education. What do we intend to do when we make moral statements? As Fr Michael Lopes OP, the coordinator of the Aids ministry of the archdiocese of San Francisco, said at the Spode conference: "A lot of our discussions of moral theology are attempts to excuse ourselves from being involved." Aids causes hysteria because it touches on two areas of human experience that cause fear—sex and death. Faced with sex and death it is easy for morality to take refuge from these painful realities. Much that is perceived of as morality may be the flight from chaos.

At the heart of our ministry to people with Aids must be the realisation that not only do we need education, but we must also allow them to educate us. Any service to the sick is not merely a matter of us bringing Christ to others but of meeting him in them. Christ always encounters us in people in need. Jesus tells us that we must clothe the naked, feed the hungry, and care for the sick, because "as you did it to one of the least of these my brethren, you did me" (Mt 25.40). The first words he spoke to the Samaritan woman at the well, and almost his last words on the cross, were "I thirst". As every priest knows, Christian care for the sick is an encounter with the Christ who is thirsty and ill. It is among the dying on the streets of Calcutta that Mother Teresa finds the body of Christ.

Fr Lopes told us during the conference about the shock of discovering Christ in a young man in an Aids ward: "After I had given him the sacraments, he lifted himself up from the bed and I gave him the Kiss of Peace. I held him in my arms and ran my hand down his back. I could feel all these lesions on his back and it was a moment of great pain for me. It became very evident to me at that moment that I was holding the Body of Christ. Then, I knew what Our Lady felt when she took the Lord's body from the cross." These words may shock us, but it is the shock of discovering what we must know if we are to serve people with Aids.

Yet we may find ourselves blocked by that old enemy of true

religion, fear. It is still the case that most people in England who have Aids are homosexual, and many people find that the encounter with homosexuality fills them with panic and disgust. Homophobia, the fear of homosexuality, is common and may even be increasing because of Aids. If one is afflicted with this phobia it is important to recognise that it is a distorted perception, a prejudice. It may make it almost impossible for one to participate directly in the Aids ministry. One may have every desire to help, and be able to support the work with prayer and financial generosity, and yet recognise that this blindness blocks us from working more closely with many Aids sufferers.

There is also the fear of sickness and death. Benedict Carter, who died of Aids in March 1987, recognised this fear in himself: "Even when I go into the Thomas Macauley Ward in St Stephen's Hospital and see an Aids patient who is very ill, I draw back and say 'Oh my God'—and I'm someone who is suffering from the illness himself. So I can appreciate what it is like for someone who is healthy." Yet in trying to care for and cherish people with Aids, we can be liberated of our fears. As Fr Michael Lopes said, "I believe it is absolutely necessary for the Church to be exposed to Aids for our own healing".

Listening without judgment

It has been estimated that at any time there are approximately one hundred times more people who are HIV-positive than have developed ARC or Aids. Once they discover that they are infected, these normal and otherwise healthy people must bear the burden of knowing that there is a high chance that they will develop a terminal illness and die within a short time. What can the Church do for them? We cannot do much alone. We must work with existing organisations, the local sexually transmitted disease clinics, the Terrence Higgins Trust and so on, so that we can identify the patients' real needs and be trained to respond to them. Dr Geraldine Mulleady, of St Mary's Hospital, Paddington, explained at the November conference that the shock of discovering that they are HIV-positive may make it difficult for people to realise that they have not actually got Aids. They may well be tempted to give up and wait to die, to let go of their lives and become passive. In this state, someone may well turn to the Church for reassurance and support and it would be scandalous if it were not easily and immediately available. We must make it as simple as possible for any Christian to discover where help is to be found. Whatever befriending or counselling services are established, nationally or locally, must be widely advertised in the Christian, medical and gay press, at the back of churches, and in sexually transmitted disease clinics.

There is no way, however, that the Church can offer any pastoral help unless we have emptied from our own minds any lingering suspicion that God may be using this illness to punish anyone. As always, good pastoral work is inseparable from good theology. When Benedict Carter first discovered he had Aids, he longed to find a priest who would simply listen, but he held back for a long time out of the dread of meeting condemnation:

> The first thing is to listen. Because I hear from people in the same condition as myself the constant complaint that "They will not listen"—and they mean the doctors and the priests, particularly the priests. I found it impossible, when I was diagnosed, to go to the Sacrament of Reconciliation because—and it might have been a copout—I said, "I've got to find a priest who understands, because to be confronted by someone who condemns one, makes one feel even more shunned and rejected, and who will turn around and say 'Go out, go away and change your whole lifestyle, otherwise I am not going to give you this free gift', that would be terrible".

Listening without judgment, learning to hear just what is said, may seem to some like a flight from morality, the renunciation of the Church's mission to teach virtue. But it is not. It is only an end to the morality that is born of a fear of the unknown, the terror of chaos. To hear without judgment is the beginning of grace, the cherishing of God's children. It is learning to hear the Christ who speaks to us through the sick and needy.

New gifts and new ministries

In the Body of Christ there are many ministries, and a new crisis can disclose new gifts. Not only can we be healed by people who are HIV-positive or who have Aids, but they can heal each other. As Dr Charles Farthing of St Stephen's Hospital, Fulham, told the Spode conference: "If you are HIV-positive and a Catholic, then I'd say that there was no better person to counsel you than someone who is HIV-positive and a Catholic". This new ministry of the sick was beautifully illustrated by Benedict Carter, who, at the Spode conference and during the remaining months of his life, was prepared to talk openly and share his experiences. He made of his suffering a preaching. The Revd Martin Hazell, of the Terrence Higgins Trust, has suggested that

118

instead of seeing gay people as a problem, we should see that they too have a special ministry in this crisis: "Gay people know what it is like to be rejected by society. . . Now if you have been able to cope with that rejection then you have something to offer. This disease is going to affect everyone. It does not matter what your sexual orientation is, whether you take drugs or not—you may yourself be rejected, whoever you are."

Yet we must also remember that service to people with Aids is not a "gay ministry" as such. In the first place, an increasing percentage of people who are HIV-positive are not homosexual but have come into contact with the virus through taking drugs, or through heterosexual sex or blood transfusion, and it is an added burden for them if Aids is thought of as the "gay plague". But secondly, even if the person is gay, the Church's ministry is not to him or her alone, but to the whole network of people who love and care for them. Fr Michael Lopes said of his pastoral visiting: "When I walk into a room, there is a chance that he is not alone. He has either a lover, or friends or his mother at his side, and brothers and sisters and a father. And the ministry that I try to do is to the whole system, to all the people there."

We cannot, by ourselves, supply all the needs of someone who is infected or ill, but we can try to help and support those who can, by reconciling people to their families and helping the people who love them. Whatever we think of the morality of a homosexual having a lover, this love may mean more to the sick or infected person than anything else at the moment. As love, it is to be celebrated as good, and it is likely to come under heavy strain at this time. Any attempt to subvert or demand that it be renounced may be to take from someone the most important support that he has. We cannot care for people unless we care for those for whom they care.

There is a growing practice of celebrating Mass to the sick and their families. "Eucharist" means, literally, thanksgiving, and if a family has been shocked by the revelation that their child is infected with Aids, then the Eucharist may offer the healing of discovering that they can give thanks with and for their child. The Eucharist was born in the face of death. Confronted with his death, Jesus took bread and broke it and gave it to his disciples, saying, "This is my body given for you". Faced with the apparent absurdity and pointlessness of his murder, this was his gesture, and it is given to us to repeat it in the face of every death, our own and that of our friends.

Aids is a highly debilitating condition. When people develop it they usually wish to remain at home as long as possible and receive hospital treatment as outpatients. But this is only possible if they are helped with all sorts of basic tasks like the cooking, the laundry, getting the shopping, keeping the place clean. And it is here that the parish has so much to offer. We should stress, said Stephen Weaver, a seminarian from Allen Hall, at the conference, "an organised lay ministry to the sick as an important group in the parish rather than emphasise an Aids ministry. We are not concerned with Aids ministries but with developing the manpower and facilities that are already present in parish communities and seeing how Aids sufferers can be included as sensitively and generously as possible".

Here, a word of caution: we must be very aware of the tension between our desire to "normalise" Aids, to treat the sufferers just as ordinary sick people, and the vital importance of respecting confidentiality. The public fear of Aids is such that even the disclosure that someone is HIV-positive can have disastrous consequences. So any offer of help from the parish must include an acute sensitivity to the act of trust someone is making when they admit to us that they have Aids. Part of ensuring that they retain a sense of control over their lives is a respect for their decision on just how public the knowledge should be. Bearing in mind these constraints, every parish can pray for people with Aids, remember them in their bidding prayers, ensure that communion is taken to them, share the chalice with them. We can also pray for the people who work with the sick, for the scientists who are trying to find a cure, for their families and the people whom they love. Prayer may look like a substitute for action, a second-best. But it is not, for it is the testimony of our belief in the God who redeems all human suffering.

If you have Aids, then the attempt to go on living an ordinary life is necessary but may be exhausting. It can also be a strain on the people with whom you live. Another of the things the Church can offer is hospitality. Parishioners' homes, and especially religious communities, can offer a place to go away and rest, to be at peace in the knowledge that one will be accepted without question or judgment. Information needs to be collected on which religious communities or homes can offer this resource.

There is enormous willingness in the Church to respond to the crisis of Aids with compassion and sensitivity. It could be a moment of healing for the whole Body of Christ. But the working party on Aids, which met after the Spode conference, concluded that our response will only be effective if it is coordinated nationally. Of course, this stands in a certain tension with our desire to see Aids as just another illness. Is this succumbing to the hysteria that is creating the crisis in the first place? I think not. We shall have to work very hard as a Church to overcome the deep fears that afflict most people faced with an illness associated so deeply with sex and death. This crisis is an invitation for us to meet Christ and be healed of terror and prejudice. As a Church, we offer people many words, words of moral exhortation, even words about the Christ who cares for the needy, forgives sinners and touches lepers. But no-one will listen to our words unless they see us do something.

18 | Aids and the prison apostolate

Richard Atherton

Principal Roman Catholic chaplain
at the Home Office

Prison walls, however sturdy, are obviously no protection against the menace of Aids. Indeed, it might be argued that the prison community constitutes one of the most vulnerable sections of the whole population, for at least three reasons. First of all, because it is made up largely of people from the most sexually active age group: more than 50 per cent of them are below the age of 30. Secondly, many have pursued a lifestyle which has made them particularly at risk where the Aids virus is concerned. And, thirdly, a large percentage of prisoners are cooped up in shared accommodation for long hours on end: at present there are more than 18,000 prisoners who are lodged two or three to a cell originally intended for one person.

The director of Prison Medical Services, Dr John Kilgour, was quick to alert the prison department in early 1985 of the difficulties that penal establishments could expect to face in the coming months and years. At the same time he offered guidelines (since revised) for dealing with inmates who are either symptomless carriers of the HIV virus, who are suffering from ARC or from "full-blown" Aids.

The prison chaplains realised that the presence of Aids among prisoners, and the certain rise in its incidence, also called for a response from them. Accordingly, three chaplains were deputed to "specialise" in this area: to develop their knowledge, to exchange information with experienced individuals or groups, and to become a resource for the chaplaincy as a whole, providing information and acting as advisors to chaplains who seek their help. They took part in a two-day intensive workshop at St Mary's Hospital, Paddington, and one has visited the United States to learn from chaplains who already have extensive first-hand experience of the pastoral care of prisoners with Aids.

By the end of March 1987, one prisoner in this country had died of Aids; he was transferred to a National Health Service Hospital before death. Another 75 had been diagnosed HIV-positive. Without doubt, many more are virus carriers but are either unaware of being ill or unwilling to reveal their condition for fear of discrimination. It is to be expected that our pastoral strategy will develop as, on the one hand, the Aids virus makes further inroads on the prison population and, on the other, as we build upon our own growing experience. However, whatever future refinements there may be, the general pattern of our pastoral work seems clear. It will extend first to prison staff, second, to the families of prisoners who are suffering from Aids or Aids-related illnesses and third, and most importantly, to the Aids patients themselves.

Upholding the dignity of Aids patients

The prison chaplain has always been regarded as chaplain not only to the prisoners but to the whole prison community. He has his own contribution to make within the interdisciplinary field of Aids, with its medical, emotional, psychological and ethical dimensions. He must be ready to cooperate with the medical and other staff who are most closely involved with caring for people with Aids. In some circumstances he may be the person best able to offer support to other carers, which is vital if they are to be sustained in an extremely stressful situation. At the same time the chaplain must recognise his own need for support, which ideally he will receive from other members of the chaplaincy team—there is an Anglican, Methodist and Roman Catholic chaplain in every penal institution—though it may come from

122

other members of staff, or from the Christian community outside. The chaplain's second task is to have sufficient understanding of the disease to be able to counter the prejudices, the ungrounded fears and anxieties, and even the open hostility which can so easily flourish in a closed society which feels itself threatened by the Aids virus. The dangers are clear from an incident in Auburn Prison, New York, where after three prisoners died of Aids one hundred inmates went on hunger-strike and demanded that all homosexuals and HIV carriers should be banned from working in the kitchens[1]. The chaplain can help to bring a sense of proportion to the situation and so allay fears, dissipate panic and reduce the risk of discrimination against prisoners with Aids.

Closely allied to this task is that of upholding the human dignity of people with Aids. The well-publicised photograph of Mr Norman Fowler shaking hands with a patient dying of Aids has perhaps done more to destigmatise Aids and to dispel unreasonable fears about the disease than all the other publicity about Aids put together. The chaplain by his whole manner of dealing with patients in the prison community—his courtesy towards them, his way of talking about them, his readiness to help them—is using the powerful language of action to say that these men and women are his fellow human beings: more than that, they are brothers and sisters "for whom Christ died" and are therefore dearly loved by God.

An intermediary with the family

The chaplain may also have pastoral responsibilities to people outside the prison, in particular to the relatives and friends of a prisoner with Aids. They will often share the same emotions as their loved one who is sick: disbelief, horror, shame, fear, anger and so on. There have in fact been some cases where a prisoner has been abandoned by his family—no more letters, no more visits—once they learned that he had been diagnosed HIV-positive. The prison chaplain may be able to fulfil a valuable role, in some cases, as an intermediary between the prisoner and his or her family, perhaps by breaking the news to them, by counselling them, or—particularly when the true condition of the prisoner is known to no-one outside except his family—by acting as confidant and friend.

However, the chief pastoral challenge facing the chaplain is to help the Aids sufferers themselves, to allow something of the unconditional love and compassion of God to flood the grim situation, to bring alive for them those words of Jesus: "Anyone who follows me will not walk in darkness, but will have the light of life" (Jn 8.12). This task will need much time and patience, but it will be close to the heart of his ministry in prison. A person with Aids is, at the present stage of medical knowledge, a person who might be described as being under sentence of death. He or she can be expected therefore to display the classical emotional responses of the dying as described by Kübler-Ross. The first reaction may well be that of disbelief ("It can't happen to me"), denial ("There's been a mistake"); but very soon it is likely to turn to anger: anger at the former associates through whom the disease was contracted; anger at the doctors and the health service because they have not found a cure; anger at God himself because he allows all this to happen.

One of the most valuable things a chaplain can do is to simply sit with the patient or carrier and allow him or her to vent the anger and hostility—which of course at times may be directed at the chaplain himself—as well as the other deep emotions of fear, loneliness and anxiety. Sooner or later anger will give place to guilt and depression: guilt for the past way of life, for "sinfulness", for the condition of associates whom he or she may have infected, guilt for the anguish caused to the family. This would seem to be the ideal time for the chaplain to lead the patient gently forward to meet Jesus in the healing and liberating encounter of the sacrament of reconciliation.

A spirit of responsibility

A great danger for the person with Aids is that in loneliness and near despair he or she will lose all interest in other people and in life itself. One young man returned from home leave in a state of great agitation, having just learned that his girlfriend was dying of Aids. He demanded that he be tested for the virus and warned the chaplain that if the test turned out positive he would "top" himself. The test proved negative, but his initial reaction highlights the overwhelming sense of despair that can be experienced by those who even suspect that they have the disease. In the United States, the expression "sheet sign" has been coined to describe the condition of people with Aids who try to escape from reality by hiding under the bedclothes[2]. The chaplain can help to head off this situation by encouraging a spirit of responsibility in the carrier or patient. "Responsibility" is a word usually taken to mean duty, but in this context it is understood in its literal sense—the "ability" to "make a response", the ability therefore to choose[3]. It is the kind of attitude so beautifully described by Fr John Dalrymple when he shows how the Christian is called to struggle by every means in his power against sickness, suffering and disease, and yet be ready at the end to bow grace-fully to God's will[4]. The person suffering from Aids still has it in his power to choose how he will face up to his fears, his anger, his failing powers, his loneliness, and ultimately his death.

To make choices, to take charge of one's life—even when it is hanging by a thread, so to say—is particularly difficult for those who have low self-esteem. Many Aids patients fall into that category because of the social stigma attached to their illness, but for prisoner-sufferers the situation is even more difficult. Already most of them have a pitifully low self-image: after all, they are society's outcasts, locked away by bolts and bars; but now they have become outcasts twice over—not simply prisoners but prisoners-with-Aids. However, the pathos of their condition makes a special appeal to the pastoral heart of the chaplain. Already, in the course of his ordinary duties, he has often been reminded that he is privileged to serve "the least of his brethren", and with that realisation comes the resolve to do everything he can to uphold the dignity of these men and women; perhaps not so much by his words but, as indicated earlier, by all of his actions.

He comes to them not simply as counsellor but as priest. Through prayer, through the Word of God, through the sacraments—the absolution that sets free, the oil that soothes and strengthens, the Bread that brings the living companionship of Jesus even to those who "walk in the valley of the shadow of death"—through these means the chaplain is able to succour the Aids patient to the end of his journey.

There was a time when every prison chaplain had to be ready to assist those who were condemned to death by execution. Times have changed, but he is still the only priest who can tell his "parishioner" who suffers from a terminal illness: "Remember, my friend, that it was to a prisoner, and to a prisoner in the very act of dying, that Jesus gave that magnificent assurance: 'This day thou shalt be with me in Paradise' (Lk 23.43)". Like the condemned cell of old, the cell of the prisoner with Aids is not the end of the story, it is simply the end of the beginning.

1. Neil Deuchar, "Aids in New York City with particular reference to the psycho-social aspects", *British Journal of Psychiatry* (1984), p. 615.

2. Ibid.
3. Antony Grey, "Aids: a counselling response", *Counselling*, No 59, Feb 1987, p. 10.
4. John Dalrymple, *Letting go in Love*, (Darton, Longman and Todd 1986).

19 | The hospital chaplain: an instrument of peace

John Arnold

Roman Catholic chaplain at Westminster Hospital

It must be said from the outset that there is no "new" challenge to the hospital chaplain in attending to the sufferers of Aids. The hospital chaplain has the duty and the privilege of being a Christian presence to the sick. He visits them simply because they are sick and he meets them as individuals. But the simplicity of this answer bears investigation and careful consideration.

To begin with, there is no question of judging anyone because of the sickness that they have, or how that sickness was contracted. At various times in recent medical history, society has seen some diseases resulting from behaviour—this person has lung cancer because she was a heavy smoker; that person has had a heart attack because he deliberately maintained a lifestyle and diet that endangered him. The hospital chaplain has never turned away from a bedside because he thought that the patient was at fault. The chaplain sees only the person as an individual and he comes to them for Christ. The basic concept underlying his task is that he should be at the bedside and act as Christ would act in those circumstances. There can be no less care and compassion for the homosexual than for the haemophiliac.

If we start from the premise that all the sick have an equal right to the chaplain's time and that the chaplain cannot distinguish between them because of the disease they have, then we can go on to consider the skills and gifts used by the chaplain which will be of particular benefit to patients who suffer from Aids.

126

First of all, and as a preliminary to almost everything else, the chaplain should attempt to bring an atmosphere of tranquillity and peace to the bedside. It is this quality which Christ carried with him throughout his ministry, which was evident within him and which he wished for those around him. Everyone in hospital is vulnerable to fear and anxiety whether they are admitted for brief and routine treatment or for a long and eventually terminal illness. They are afraid of the unknown and anxious about losing full health and mobility. Generally speaking this fear is likely to be more powerful the more serious the illness. For Aids patients, their fear and anxiety may be highly developed since, for the foreseeable future at least, the condition is terminal and the tragedy is heightened because they are generally young. For many, there is not just the question of overcoming fear for themselves, difficult enough in itself, but anxiety at the reaction of family, sexual partners and friends. There are other problems that arise of stigma and guilt, sometimes bitterness on the part of patients and a feeling of betrayal on the part of their families.

There has been fear about Aids among doctors, nurses and domestic staff in the hospitals, though these have been reduced by in-service training and excellent articles in medical journals. Careless, not to say reckless, misinformation in the media has also contributed to a near state of panic. While anyone may be an instrument of peace at the bedside of a patient, the chaplain especially has this duty and privilege in the face of fear.

Peace in the face of fear

Three elements should be cultivated in the life of the chaplain in order to maintain this peace upon which an untold number of people rely. In the first place, the chaplain should inform himself about the disease in order to be able to expel the many myths that panic and ignorance have conjured up. It is important, for example, that he should know that "barrier nursing"—which involves certain measures of isolation and the use of sterilised equipment—is not required for Aids patients, and that handshakes and embraces are not dangerous. If the chaplain appears to be unsure of what precautions are necessary in any given case, his uneasiness can easily be communicated to the patient and increase what may already be a pronounced feeling of isolation and loneliness. When the chaplain talks to those who are caring for the patients, or to their families or friends, the right information may easily help to allay fears and suspicions.

The chaplain must also be at peace with himself about the various moral questions surrounding homosexuality and drug abuse if he is to bring peace to others. It has already been powerfully stated elsewhere that "the bedside of a gay Aids patient is not the place for the pastor to be working out his or her anxieties about sexuality"[1].

Finally, to promote the peace that the chaplain should carry with him, there must be prayer. True peace comes from Christ alone, channelled by the faith of the chaplain. There can be no substitute for a chaplain's prayer for the people in his care, for through it he becomes an instrument in God's hands and his own human efforts are strengthened by grace. It must surely be the experience of every chaplain that the good that is done goes beyond human capability—God is at work despite the shortcomings of those who are his instruments.

Beyond words, the sacraments

Meanwhile, the importance of the sacraments always goes beyond words and actions. The priest in the hospital makes frequent use of three sacraments: the Eucharist, Reconciliation, and Anointing of the Sick. They must often be introduced with care and sensitivity since the fear of anointing as Extreme Unction is by no means past. The very presence of a priest in the ward may suggest to some that death is not very far away. The chaplain must make it clear to all that his work is for the most part a visiting of all those in hospital who would appreciate it, no matter how ill or near to recovery they are.

The idea that a priest comes only to give the last rites may well be in the mind of the Aids patient because he or she is aware of the terminal nature of the illness. Most Aids sufferers know, however, that the disease does not usually progress rapidly and that a considerable time may elapse before its final stages.

Another barrier between the chaplain and the Aids patient may occur, however, because of the perception that people with Aids belong to a group which has been roundly condemned by the Church. Only through personal contact may the chaplain allay these fears. What the Church has said is "disordered" in homosexuality is the activity itself; it does not condemn the individuals themselves. In the same way, drug abuse is condemned but not the people who use the drugs. The Church must be able to speak on moral issues, but it must never close the doors on individuals. Christ spoke clearly about morality and he condemned immoral practices, but never did he write anyone off because they indulged in these things. On the contrary, he sought them out, forgave them and taught them. The chaplain can do no other. To those who distrust the Church or who feel bitterness the chaplain must simply make himself available and make it known that he has no agenda other than to offer time and friendship.

If the opportunity begins to present itself, then the use of the sacraments may become an important part of the chaplain's relationship with the patient. Progress achieved by the patient's counsellor, or by friends and other helpers, may well be strengthened by reception of the Eucharist or by Reconciliation.

Not a counsellor

One thing that the chaplain must keep firmly in mind is that he is not himself a counsellor, in the sense now given to the term in psycho-medical practice. To assume such a role would be mistaken for two reasons. In the first place, counselling requires a great amount of time, which the chaplain in the ordinary course of his ministry does not have. There will surely be occasions when a patient requires a great deal of time, particularly during the final stages of a terminal illness, but normally it is neither appropriate or possible for the chaplain to give sufficient attention to each patient to undertake counselling. In the second place, the priest, unless specifically trained, does not have the various sophisticated skills required. Counselling is more than simply listening and showing compassion. The chaplain who embarks on counselling another, without the required training, is likely to do harm rather than good.

There is a further danger in the chaplain assuming the role of a counsellor, for it can easily blur his essential role as a befriender in Christ, who brings the presence of the Church and her sacraments to the patient. The counsellor tries to put the patient in touch with himself or herself, and to acknowledge and confront problems which may or may not have their roots in questions of faith or spirituality. If the chaplain attempts this process, confusion may result for the patient, and prove an obstacle to spiritual peace of mind, since all problems could so easily be thought to stem from religious experience. Trained counsellors who are priests are most careful to distinguish the spiritual from the non-spiritual and the hospital chaplain may unwittingly confuse this distinction.

Dr James Hanratty, of St Joseph's Hospice in Hackney, has

written about the terminal stages, the "last 48 hours" of an illness. In fact, this may last one or two hours or a week. But, whatever the length, it is a distinct, final and separate stage. Dr Hanratty says that at this stage the patient should never be left alone. Normally, of course, there will be friends and relatives with a patient, but at this more than at any other time, there must be a sense of peace and the simple support of someone's physical presence.

For the patient, the last hours are often a time of heightened awareness in certain matters. While oblivious to much that may be happening, details such as a soothing word, a prayer, or a hand being held may create a strong peace of mind.

Preparing for bereavement

For family and friends, these last hours are of great importance because they will be so clearly remembered in the coming months and it helps the period of bereavement if this time is peaceful for all. The nursing staff and the doctors are chiefly responsible for creating an atmosphere of calm as well as for medical treatment at this stage. It is important that the patient—insofar as it is possible—and visitors should know what the medical staff are doing and why.

At this stage, the chaplain may well be directly involved in administering the sacraments, or he may simply be present at the bedside. There may be things to be said but frequently there is little or no need for conversation and the chaplain should be sensitive to whether or not others wish to speak. Prayers often provide a necessary escape from a need to talk, and almost always prayers speaking of the love and forgiveness of God and the peace of the life to come are welcomed and appreciated.

In the terminal stages of Aids, a particular sickness such as cancer or pneumonia becomes predominant. This highlights the basic truth that the Aids patient is simply another person with a sickness whose final hours are to be made as comfortable and as peaceful as possible, in a medical and spiritual sense.

Bereavement also has its own unique expression in every case. More often than not, this is a process which occurs away from the hospital and out of reach of the chaplain. But he should make the offer to friends and relatives to stay in touch: this may be all he can do, although the bereavement process may be helped if he is asked to conduct the funeral of a patient.

There is nothing new in the challenge of Aids to the hospital chaplain. True, the patient and his or her family may feel the

sense of guilt and stigma that are attached to the illness. It is also
tragic that most of the victims are young, and their death carries
its own particular distress. But the chaplain uses the same
sensitivity and offers his own very limited presence to people
with Aids as to anyone else. In return, he will have those
moments when he knows that what he has brought to the
bedside—whether sacramentally or in friendship—has been of
importance. At other times he will not know whether anything
has been achieved or he may be faced with rejection, for
whatever reason. While the challenge is not new, Aids offers a
reminder of the enormity of the challenge which faces the
Christian community to prepare, and help others to prepare,
with dignity and maturity, for the inevitability of death. No
matter in what circumstances we arrive at the end of our lives
we should be reminded of the love of God, his infinite mercy and
of his longing for us to be reconciled with him.

1. Aids: some guidelines for pastoral care (Church House Publishing, 1986).

20 | When a friend has Aids

James Hanvey SJ
A doctoral student at Campion Hall, Oxford, who spent
the summer of 1986 working with the Aids/ARC
programme of the archdiocese of San Francisco

Especially through his lifestyle and through his actions, Jesus
revealed that love is present in the world in which we live—an
effective love, a love that addresses itself to man and
embraces everything that makes up his humanity. This love
makes itself particularly noticed in contact with suffering,
injustice and poverty—in contact with the whole historical
"human condition", which in various ways manifests man's
limitation and frailty, both physical and moral.
Dives in Misericordia

"What is the person with Aids looking for from the Church?"
This seems like a good question, the sort that any concerned
person might ask. I have heard it put by many people who

feel that their faith requires some personal response to the present crisis of Aids. Occasionally, it is asked by priests and religious or by bishops and church administrators, who are often under pressure to produce statements or devise strategies. They are conscious that Aids is yet another area of modern existence where life seems to outstrip and expose the limitations of our neat conceptual frameworks, whether they are moral, political or theological. It was also the question originally suggested as a basis for this article.

However, this may be the first question, but there is another which must take priority. And that is: Are you really open to the answer?

If, as individuals or as a community, we have not asked *this* question of ourselves, then we run the risk of a response which is only an exercise in public relations or the shallow pragmatism of crisis management, lasting only as long as the media decides or public attention permits.

"Are you really open to the answer?" questions the basis on which we come to people with Aids. Without doubt we come with all the usual good intentions, thinking, in fact, that we have something to offer. The basis for this assumption, however, is not obvious: many agencies and groups both in this country and in America recognised the crisis long before the Christian community and are engaged in deeply committed, generous and compassionate service purely on the basis of human need. They work freely and openly, without any of the prejudices and the extraordinarily complex manoeuvres that Churches and hierarchies feel they must go through.

A modern road to Emmaus

Although it is clear that Aids is not a "gay" disease, in America and in Europe at present the majority of people with Aids or ARC are homosexual. It is had to avoid the impression that the Catholic Church is, at least, embarrassed by this; a reaction often compounded by the fact that Aids inevitably raises questions about sexual mores and practices. The Church seems to find it difficult to separate the suffering and need of the person with Aids from his or her previous lifestyle. Indeed, many who have the disease will already have experienced hostility and alienation from the Church community.

The further question which must therefore be addressed to the Church or anyone with a desire to help is: "How committed are you to those who have this disease?"

132

It is clear that there will be no sudden cure and in many forms Aids, with all its related problems, will be with society for a long time to come. Will you be there in the long nights and routine days as people with Aids try to maintain life as well as face death? Will you still be there with their families and friends, still prepared to develop the necessary human, spiritual and material resources? When all the panic and the paranoia has died away and public attention has moved on to something else, will you still be there with those who have Aids or ARC?

We have evidence that there is a deep desire among many Christians to say "yes" to all these questions; to set out on this strange modern road to Emmaus: the paradigm journey of all the Church's pastoral ministry. Yet the journey has its conditions:

Openness to learning

Unlike most journeys there is no predetermined destination. There is just the hope that something of the love of Christ will appear along the way. It is a journey which cannot have the security of answers in advance and therefore all who make it must be ready to learn. Learning means that we must be prepared to listen and this is not always easy for a Church which is used to giving answers and is often under pressure from people to supply them.

Openness to listening

Listening is the first action of love for its focus is on the one who is suffering and in need. It is also a listening for the way in which the Spirit is moving through a person's life and experience. As with any sickness, not least with Aids, the real teachers are those who are ill and unless we are prepared to recognise this we have nothing to give but our own prejudices and our tired, safe cliches. The prerequisite for all of this is the humility which comes from freedom—the freedom to meet another person on his or her ground, to accept a situation in which there are contradictions, in which all the forms of "ego", whether personal or ecclesiological, have to be left aside. It is a freedom from the tyranny of moral, social or political respectability. In the end it is the freedom to set out in search of Christ, allowing him to choose the place where he will meet us. It is also the freedom of Christ in his Crucifixion. If we are not prepared for that then we have no place in this work for we will only

133

contribute to the hurt, the frustration and the alienation of those who have the disease; we will only be adding our own needs and preoccupations to an agenda which is already too full.

The capacity for conversion

When we ask how we can help, are we prepared for the answer: Conversion—a change of heart?

> Conversion is the most concrete expression of the working of love and of the presence of mercy in the human world. The true and proper meaning of mercy does not consist only in looking, however penetratingly and compassionately, at moral, physical or material evil: mercy is manifested in its true and proper aspect when it restores to value, promotes and draws good from all the forms of evil existing in the world and man.
> *Dives in Misericordia*

Only if we are willing to allow the Spirit to work in us in this way by calling us beyond the security of our institutions and our categories towards persons can we have something worthy to offer.

The first effect of this will be to change our question to "What do we do when a friend has Aids?" When that is our question, we may have discovered the richness of our own life as Christian; we may have discovered here, with those we never saw or cared about before, the source of the Church's life: "You are my friends" (Jn 15.14).

This is the reality of the work of grace: God's free and unmerited gift of himself to us who also need healing. For when a friend has Aids all you can do, all you need to do, is to love graciously.

The sacrament of our humanity

> . . . it will be good to call attention to two points:
>
> 1. The first is that love ought to manifest itself in deeds rather than words.
>
> 2. The second is that love consists in a mutual sharing of goods, for example, the one who loves gives and shares with the one loved what he possesses, or something that he has or is able to give. . . . Thus one always gives to the other.
> Prelude to *Contemplatio Ad Amorem*
> St Ignatius of Loyola, Sp. Exx. 231

Aids is not a "gay" disease, an "African" disease or one that belongs to intravenous drug users. It is a *human* disease. People with Aids are of every class and type, some with many personal, social and spiritual resources, others with very few. Their friends, parents and families also have questions, fears and needs. It is in this situation that the Christian community can offer its own rich resource of love and healing—it does have a ministry. It is the Spirit's imperative to walk with all those who are abandoned and alienated whether through suffering and debilitating illness or through moral, political or economic oppression (*Gaudium et Spes 1; Mt 25.11ff*). Although in many cases these people will find themselves on the fringes of the institution they are never on the fringes of the Church: indeed, they are at its heart.

Love must be practical if it is to be real. Aids, like any fatal or debilitating illness, robs us of ourselves. It is not just the physical humiliation or the anxiety, it is the need to know that we are still of worth and still loveable. There is no unrealistic expectation of some sudden cure, there is simply the need for the really important things—friendship, company, humour and hope—the hope that you still matter to someone. Above all it is the need to know that you are not alone, that you can share all the questions, fears and anger as well as the grace and sometimes the fun. The first sacrament is the sacrament of our humanity and it is found in all the ordinary, routine things. It is found in the just being there through the long nights, in a touch, a smile or a kiss; it is found in the fact that even with Aids life still goes on in all its mundane activity and not so divine comedy. When a friend has Aids to be practical means that you first have to be there—the sacrament of presence. Anyone who loves can be its minister; no-one is excluded from it and it is unconditional.

An opportunity to think again

As in any situation which raises fundamental questions, it is not only the person who has Aids who is challenged to reflect upon the meaning of his or her life and its values. Those who care for them, the Church and society, will also have to reflect. Often caricatures and assumptions, phobias and prejudices which are very deep-seated will have to be left behind. It is also the time to rediscover values which we may have forgotten or the power in virtues which social fashions and theories had claimed were obsolete. The articulate prophets of sexual liberalism may well have proved false. Aids presents us with an opportunity to think

135

again, to grow and perhaps reach a new maturity in the things that matter. It may be offering us an opportunity to create a Church and a community in which people do not need to disguise or lie about what they are as if they had been branded with some mark of Cain. It gives us the possibility of creating a Church in which people can live in the truth and with the truth, accepted and valued for their humanity. Aids confronts us with our blindness and offers us all a time for healing. Really practical caring will not try to avoid these deeper and more radical dimensions by taking refuge in some sort of doctrine of "moral neutrality" or benign pragmatism because such an approach is also, in the end, dehumanising and alienating.

Of course those who have Aids and ARC also have their own prejudices and assumptions. There are those who have contracted Aids through intravenous drug abuse and take some sort of moral refuge in the thought that "at least I'm not queer". There are some who may want to portray themselves as victims of a hostile society and those who find it difficult to accept responsibility for their own lives and actions. Whatever the circumstances, there is no-one who does not need understanding and acceptance, if not approval.

The isolation of priests with Aids

Within this wide and complex spectrum, there is perhaps one small group which calls for our special attention: priests and religious who have Aids. They are in a particularly isolated position. Given that the principal way in which Aids is transmitted is through sexual contact with an infected person, the whole integrity and moral life of a priest or religious person with Aids will be under scrutiny and exposed to public judgment. Often, for prudent and not necessarily punitive reasons, bishops and superiors have tried to avoid scandal and publicity. At times the way in which this has been handled has seemed lacking in compassion. A priest or religious with Aids is perhaps one of the most isolated and vulnerable members of the community. He will have deep and painful questions to face in the solitude of his own heart and conscience. Yet by vocation he belongs to the community and it cannot abandon him or pretend that he does not exist. Here the words of the prophets have special power:

> But Zion said, "The Lord has forsaken me, my Lord has forgotten me." Can a woman forget her sucking child, that

136

she should have no compassion on the son of her womb? Even these may forget, yet I will not forget you (Is 49.14–15).

At the heart of priesthood is an austere and profound beauty. It is the sacrament of service which can only be realised though a deep self-emptying, a *kenosis* in the name and image of Christ. It is for this reason that the sacrament belongs to the very *being* of the person. It becomes the form and the horizon of his life and its meaning. As such it has an eternal reality before God and in the community of his people and it is never just a matter of function. Yet it is also lived in the changing patterns and circumstances of a human life. Even in frailty and brokenness and priest never loses his power to minister and indeed those very conditions may lead him to new ways of service.' The Church should not be ashamed to recognise this.

No-one stands alone before God

When a person has Aids he or she begins a long journey. If it is understood aright and accompanied by love it becomes a journey towards healing. The deepest level of this is reconciliation—reconciliation with the past and all the relationships and pain that have been part of the journey. It is also a reconciliation with the future: the fear of disfigurement and debilitation; the fear of losing control and dignity, but most of all the fear of being alone and once more alienated. Even at the end, there can be the fear that God may hate you the way others seem to. It is here, at this moment, that the Christian community knows the richness and depth of the gift it has been given, for the source of its life is reconciliation. Out of its own knowledge of the graciousness of the God "who has reconciled us to himself" the community shares that gift with anyone in need. The community accomplishes this not only through its concrete sacraments but through its solidarity—its gathering of all those who stand alone in their pain and doubt and fear. No-one stands alone before God; they stand as part of a community which knows them and loves them, nourishes and prays for them. Even at the moment of death the future is crowded with friends; there is always the Church that "has gone before us marked with the sign of faith", a faith which is "known to God alone".

The requirements of justice

These are some of the dimensions and aspects of showing a practical and Christ-like love when a friend has Aids. Clearly, their principal focus is on the personal. However, it would not be correct to conclude this reflection without drawing attention to another vitally important and practical action which the whole Church can carry out most effectively and precisely as a community.

Faith cannot be separated from the desire for justice. For the Christian, justice is not simply the requirement of law or a theory of political and economic structure. It is the work of Christ in his Cross and Resurrection. Justice is the work of reconciliation, the sign of the righteousness and mercy of God, a work of his love.

Aids raises questions of justice and the Church has a responsibility to speak out in the name of justice and compassion. It must speak out against the paranoia and all the phobias which threaten people's rights and would seek to deprive them of their basic dignity and privacy. Equally, it must remind individuals and groups in high-risk communities that the grace of belonging to a community also entails obligations. Those who have Aids or ARC also have the responsibility to love.

In the allocation of resources we must be aware not only of needs but of the requirements of justice. Money allocated in our society for the care of patients and research into the disease should not endanger or restrict the funds available to other programmes for the vulnerable, such as the elderly, the chronically disabled and the homeless. It may mean that once again we have to critically examine our priorities and the economic ideology which seems able to find contingency funds for military purposes but is unable to extend these to Aids.

One of the most pressing needs for those who have Aids is accommodation. Often when a person is diagnosed as HIV-positive they can come under pressure either from those they live with or landlords to move. They need "safe" accommodation where they can carry on living as normally as possible without undue attention and harassment. At some point hospices may have a part to play, but not everyone wants to use them. As the number of people with Aids increases it is unlikely that hospices would be sufficient given the other demands on them. It may be that hostels and day-centres provide a better option. The Christian community may find it has the ability to help in making these resources available.

We also know that drug abuse is not only a problem of the rich and famous. It is the young unemployed and homeless who are most at risk. If there is to be a cure for Aids then we also need to cure deprivation and expose the effects of the prevailing economic orthodoxies. We need to reexamine the sort of society they produce and assess their true cost to human beings.

So far the discussion and reflection of this article has been within the context of Aids as a Western problem. We now know that it is not and that it threatens other countries, particularly in Africa, which are much more vulnerable because they have practically no resources to meet the demands of the disease. When a friend has Aids we must not only share ourselves and our expertise but our financial and material resources as well. The demands of friendship, justice and love are as universal as the Church. Africa is a friend.

When a friend has Aids there may not be much time to undertake a lengthy reflection on all the issues. We simply have to set out on the journey. Occasionally, on the way, we may glimpse the beginning of the answer to the questions, but perhaps most of all there may be a discovery that we can leave the questions and their demands for answers behind. In taking the risk to set out, to reach beyond our own doubts and boundaries, choosing to start with the mandatum of Holy Thursday—"that you love one another as I have loved you"—even the Friday of Aids must move forward to another morning with all its hope.

PART VI | A variety of religious perspectives

21 | Time for moral renaissance

Basil Hume OSB
Cardinal Archbishop of Westminster

Some people have claimed that the Aids epidemic is God's punishment of a sinful world. It is better seen as proof of a general law that actions have consequences and that disorder inevitably damages and then destroys.

In fact, Aids is neither the whole problem nor the central issue. It is a symptom of something deeper and more deadly. Aids is but one of the many disastrous consequences of promiscuous sexual behaviour. Promiscuity is the root-cause of the present epidemic. It has always been sinful; it is rapidly becoming suicidal.

A call for greater stress on the moral issues

We are, then, dealing with an intrinsically moral issue and not simply one of public health. No campaign against Aids can ignore or trivialise the moral question. Refusal to address the moral issues is itself a moral statement.

In the public campaign so far, much attention has been focussed in very explicit terms on the way the virus has been transmitted and on precautions to reduce the risk of infection. Too little has been said so far, and too vaguely, about the radical shift in attitudes needed to halt the advance of the epidemic. Yet morality, when, as here, it concerns matters of life and death, affects the public good and involves the whole community. It is certainly not the exclusive concern of the Church and the clergy.

The Church and the government have a common aim, to limit and, if possible, eliminate the disease. The Church wants to tackle promiscuity as the principal cause of infection. I would argue that the government itself could legitimately, and helpfully, lay greater stress on the moral issues.

Reappraisal of attitudes

No purpose can be served by recriminations against any section of the population held to be responsible. Instead, we should

143

offer to those with Aids unconditional and practical compassion. It would be unfortunate, too, if reaction took the form of a merciless and self-righteous moral backlash. Something much more radical and constructive is called for than the scourging of other people's vices. If a catastrophe is to be averted there must be an urgent and immediate reappraisal of our attitudes and behaviour in matters of sexual behaviour and human relationship.

Even in the short-term a moral reawakening is society's best hope. That must be part of any national programme of information and education. Condoms and free needles for drug addicts will reduce but not remove the dangers. Those most at risk might be led to conclude that a potentially lethal lifestyle can, with precautions, be made safe.

The fact to be faced is that all of us in society have to learn to live according to a renewed set of values. That will not be easy. How can any appeal for faithfulness and sexual restraint be heeded when there is on all sides explicit encouragement to promiscuous behaviour and frequent ridicule of moral values. Society is in moral disarray for which we must all take our share of blame. Sexual permissiveness reflects the general decline of values in public and private life.

Some might question whether any consensus on values is possible in a society which has so lost touch with its cultural, religious and spiritual roots. Nonetheless, I am convinced that there are untapped reserves of goodness and idealism in many individuals and communities. Laying the foundations for a new consensus will be prolonged, arduous and quite often hotly contested.

The search for a better way, the endeavour to reconstruct society's attitudes and values will, of necessity, take many forms. Together we must reflect on the consequences of our common humanity, the needs and longings of the human heart. We can learn, too, from history while not idealising the past. There can be no question, even if it were possible, of attempting to turn back the clock. The situation we confront demands of us a new response.

The Christian Churches have an obvious part to play in this fundamental rethinking. So, too, have the world religions now represented in our country. The Judaeo-Christian heritage of moral values still has much to offer contemporary society. We can learn much also from the traditions of asceticism and self-discipline prized by Islam and the great religions of the East. Reconstruction demands serious dialogue. People, whether

144

religious or not, can surely find common ground and shared ideals in face of the manifest dangers which threaten society.

Some are prepared to concede that such a transformation is required but believe it to be a long-term objective. It is necessary in the short-term, they argue, to adopt the measures advocated in the present campaign of public education on Aids. The Roman Catholic Church in this country is being urged to modify its opposition to the use of condoms and its condemnation of sexual activity outside marriage, at least in the case of stable relationships. There are, however, serious matters of principle which the Church is not at liberty to ignore.

The Christian vision of love and marriage

Roman Catholic teaching maintains that human love is a precious gift, a sharing in the life and love of God himself. Unselfish love between persons is itself a way to God. It enriches the human personality. In married love a couple come together in a lifelong, life-giving union in which they give themselves totally and exclusively to each other. To be fully human and self-giving, that love has to remain open to the possibility of new life. It provides the stability and affection necessary for the nurturing and development of the growing child. For all these reasons, the full sexual expression of love is reserved for husband and wife within marriage.

The Roman Catholic Church, therefore, cannot be expected to lend support to any measures which tacitly accept, even if they do not encourage, sexual activity outside marriage. To do so would be inconsistent. It would weaken our primary witness to the Christian vision of human love and marriage. Nor do we accept that for the unmarried the choice lies solely between condoms and infection. There is a third course of action: refusal to engage in extra-marital sexual activity. Such self-discipline is not emotionally destructive, but can be a positive affirmation of a radical ideal, demanding but not impossible.

The Roman Catholic Church is committed to the cause of marriage and family life. It is a sad reflection on present values that no political party offers a coherent and comprehensive policy to sustain and uphold family life. Here there is much common ground to be explored. It is essential to enhance the quality of individual and family life.

A radical change in popular attitudes is possible, indeed necessary. Many in recent years have become convinced of the need to embrace a simpler, healthier lifestyle in order to enjoy

145

a fuller, longer life. We are already changing deep-rooted habits in eating, drinking, smoking, and exercise. How much greater is the necessity to rediscover the joy of faithful love and lasting marriage. It calls for self-discipline, restraint and a new awareness. Such a profound change in society also needs a comprehensive campaign of public education and persuasion.

Spirit of dialogue and hope

The Aids crisis represents a watershed for contemporary society. It is much more than a matter of sexual morality. Shared moral values derive from an accepted understanding of society. Fear may well induce some to modify their sexual behaviour. That is not enough, however, to achieve that radical renewal of society which is so clearly needed. The necessary steps should be taken, I would suggest, in an atmosphere of calm and trust and in a spirit of dialogue and hope. There is much to be done in the home, in schools and in every part of our life and work together. Parents, teachers, clergy, communicators, those in public and political life all have shared responsibility to discover new hope and a better way.

© *Times Newspapers Ltd*, 7 January 1987

22 | Facing the moral dilemmas

John Habgood
Archbishop of York

There is no one moral approach to the question of Aids: we need different approaches in different circumstances. We need a combination of practical wisdom and a concern about principle.

What one might call the principled approach to Aids as a social problem has of course received very wide publicity, and I have some sympathy with it. Undoubtedly the main means of infection have been through sexual promiscuity and drug abuse, practices which until recently have been clearly and unequivocally regarded as wrong. This has led many people to describe the whole problem in clear theological language as the judgment of God. I do not believe that the picture of a God who judges us in this way squares very well with the understanding of God that I derive from the New Testament. But there is some validity in it: there is a connection between what our society has been doing to itself and what has now come upon us.

We can also see other connections: I was intrigued by a recent letter in the *New Scientist* in which the writer was speculating on the origin of Aids, saying that it seems too much of a coincidence to suppose that HIV originated just at the very moment when conditions were ideal for its spread. It seems much more likely, the writer said, that the virus had been around for a long time but only survived in societies which were thinly populated, rural, immobile, and usually governed by strong sexual inhibitions. What has now brought the virus into prominence, and given it its hold, are the changed social conditions where we now have a close-knit population with many people who are sexually promiscuous and highly mobile; these have created the ideal conditions for the infection to escalate.

Be that as it may, whatever the interpretation placed upon it, there is a connection between the epidemic and major social and moral changes.

I personally believe that a straightforward appeal to moral principles is not going to help us much at this stage, for a number of reasons. First, as is well known in our society, not all people share the same moral principles, particularly about sexual behaviour. Secondly, even where there is broad agreement about general moral principles on sex, there has been a shift in perception. For instance, many have much more positive and accepting attitudes towards homosexuals, and on the whole most people would regard this as a moral advance rather than a retrograde step. Whatever one makes of homosexuality as such, it is not good to have a minority in our culture who feel persecuted and cut off from the mainstream; it is not good to invoke a simplistic moralism in which certain people are simply condemned for being what they are.

Thirdly, if we associate Aids too closely with moral guilt, then we are being unfair on those people who catch the disease for reasons for which they are in no way unblameworthy: for example, a girl who marries a man who has no idea that he is infected and becomes infected herself; a child infected by its mother; haemophiliacs. If the disease carries a moral stigma, then we are simply adding to the burden of suffering which these people already have to carry. Moreover, if certain people are labelled as guilty, they are not actually going to come forward to identify themselves.

The difficulties of moral persuasion

Public morality tends to be utilitarian anyway: it is a morality of consequences, not making great play with principles, but trying to look in practical ways at harmful and beneficial effects. Most public legislation has to be based on that kind of moral basis rather than on high moral principle. These, I think, are the reasons why public programmes concerned with the prevention of the spread of Aids, on the whole, carefully avoid the moral issues. But can we avoid them completely? I do not think so.

Legislation on sexually transmitted diseases has not had much success. A second approach has been through moral persuasion. One of its difficulties has been its double motivation. There was a health motivation— moral screws were put on people for the benefit of their health—but at the same time there were those who saw this as a way of improving the general climate of sexual morality. These two motives competed with and confused one another. Let me quote from a church report of 1924 which is startlingly relevant to 1987: "To say 'avoid this and you will suffer from it' is to stimulate ingenuity to find the means by which the consequences can be avoided and the act enjoyed". That is the ambiguity from the point of view of the moralist. From the point of view of the medical profession the ambiguity showed itself in that doctors felt that if they took a heavy moral line (and many of them wanted to because they saw the benefit in terms of health if they did) they were appearing judgmental. They felt they were putting a moral barrier between themselves and their patients.

So the medical profession moved to moral indifference, in effect saying, "This is not to be regarded as a moral problem at all. We can't deal with this aspect of it, so we'll treat it simply as a medical problem." I quote here from an Office of Health Economics pamphlet dated 1974: "Attempts to control sexual behaviour, preventing promiscuity and so limiting the chances of infection spreading, are unlikely to be successful and may today be thought absurd by those to whom they are directed. This area is so complex that would-be educators who try to change the population's sexual behaviour may even influence it in a manner which is the reverse of that which they intended."

But moral indifference is itself a moral attitude. Unconcern about sexual behaviour expresses the belief that it doesn't

148

matter. This conveys a positive message to others that it doesn't matter what they do. That is why, in the end, no matter how hard we try, we cannot escape making moral judgments, whether explicitly and consciously, or implicitly by what we fail to do or say. But the opposite of indifference, intolerance and moral condemnation, are not the only options. We do not need to be judgmental in caring morally and demonstrating by our attitude that we have moral standards which matter to us.

How to use our insight and concern

So it is useful to distinguish between tolerance on the one hand and indifference on the other. Indifference is saying that none of these things matter; tolerance is saying, "I may differ from you in my attitude towards your sexual behaviour but, nevertheless, I am going to tolerate you and accept you as a person and treat you as a person." It seems to me that keeping that distinction alive can enable a moral approach to develop, which is not judgmental.

In the past there has been the possibility of cure of sexually-transmitted diseases. To some extent the impersonal technical approach was justified because the disease could actually be treated. With Aids the wider social and moral questions cannot be avoided. And one of the most urgent questions is how to use our moral insight and concern as an ally in the fight against Aids without running into the dangers of simply arousing guilt and counter reactions.

My experience of joint World Council of Churches and World Health Organisation conferences indicates different stages in reaction to Aids. The first stage almost always tends to be a denial of the problem: it's somebody else's problem; it's a problem for homosexuals; it's a problem for degenerate Western society. It's too painful to see that it may be our problem, anybody's problem.

The situation is particularly agonising in Africa and it was noticeable that many of the African Church representatives at one of our meetings had a strong tendency to withdraw from the problem and say, "It doesn't really exist; the supposed figures in Africa have been exaggerated; there are only 2,000 notified cases"—flatly denying the widely canvassed estimate of tens or hundreds of thousands of cases. There is extreme sensitivity about homosexuality, which is not recognised as being part of African culture at all. Because there is no accurate estimate of the size of the problem, there is huge fear; and when faced with huge fear people run away. One of the reasons for not welcoming accurate information is that the resources to cope with infection are so scanty that to face it is too painful, in the knowledge of how little can actually be done. Even the use of clean needles for routine medical purposes is sometimes beyond the scope of some of the poorer African countries. Thus there is a search for alternative explanations: mosquitoes, tourists, etc.

In face of such attitudes and prospects, prosperous Western countries have a very strong moral obligation to help Third World countries by medical advice, supplies and know-how.

Contradictory signals

After the phase of not wanting to know, comes the phase of over-reaction, panic, feelings that Aids can be spread by almost anything. For instance, there has been much rather panicky debate in church circles about the use of the common cup in the Communion service, with many irrational and unfounded fears being expressed. It is important for those in the medical profession, and those who have a scientific background, to realise how little the public on the whole understands about the limits of certainty in science and medicine. Scientists and doctors tend to hedge their remarks by calling risks "almost negligible" or "miniscule"; but to those who are not used to such language, "almost negligible" sounds terribly threatening. Again, because we are at the stage in which the pattern of the disease is being unravelled and much is still not known, there are many contradictory signals coming from the medical profession; these cause alarm and confusion because, on the whole, the assumption is that doctors know. Whereas in many cases they do not.

Contacts with the homosexual community disclose the enormous feeling of rejection and persecution which many are suffering at the moment. One thing which the World Council of Churches has tried to do in its own statements on the subject is to stress that Aids should not be used as a basis for this kind of discrimination.

So if "not wanting to know" and panic are inappropriate reactions, what are the appropriate ones? Education, obviously. The government educational programme is not above criticism, but needs to be affirmed. The condom programme, and the programme for giving out free needles to drug addicts, seem to me to be sensible. I believe the government is wise to avoid giving out free condoms because, whereas free needles are a response to a certain kind of necessity well-recognised in the drug addict, giving out free condoms would seem a positive invitation to sexual promiscuity.

Solving the dilemmas

I wonder, though, whether a condom advertisement campaign need be quite so morally neutral. There are unresolved questions about how effective condoms are anyway. If there is a discernible failure rate in contraception when dealing with objects as large as sperm, what is the failure rate like to be when dealing with very small objects like viruses? Moreover, can a condom regime be maintained on a long-term basis without reinforcement by some more fundamental behavioural change?

But then there is a further question: how can such a behavioural change take place in a morally confused society like our own, without appealing to religious motivation, which in any case only affects a minority, or without running into all the problems of ambivalence which were obvious in the venereal disease programmes, or without provoking counter-reactions?

There is of course another range of ethical issues which particularly affect the medical profession—issues concerned with testing, whether indirectly through the case findings or through some general screening programme. What is to be done with the knowledge obtained? And what sort of pressure is put on people who learn the truth but cannot be offered any kind of cure?

I believe these moral dilemmas will only begin to be solved when it is seen that there are at least some minimal things which can be done for those who are diagnosed as being HIV-positive. Perhaps some of the palliative treatments may provide an excuse for trying to identify more infected sufferers. Support groups for Aids patients can also provide the kind of context in which there is a positive advantage in being told that one is infected and that counselling and support are available. It is a small point, but in trying to do more for those patients known to be infected, we may find that the moral issues surrounding the questions about screening become less horrific.

In an article in *The Times* in February 1987, my aim was to explore the link between intimacy and vulnerability. Intimate relations make us vulnerable, both physiologically and psychologically. Aids is now a classic example of the former. In particular, HIV attacks us at the fundamental biological level where our identity is safeguarded, namely through our immune

151

system. But intimate relationships also make us vulnerable psychologically; and this is why they are so threatening for so many people. We have to open ourselves, expose ourselves, to another person; and it is because of these vulnerabilities that intimate relationships have always, historically and in every culture, been surrounded by ceremonies, rules and taboos. Our culture has passed through a phase of throwing off many traditional inhibitions in the name of freedom. Paradoxically, in doing this we have imposed a new kind of bondage on ourselves. If all intimate relationships are reduced to sexual relationships, if it is impossible to be secure in relationships with other people without the risk of them turning into sexual ones, human life has been diminished rather than expanded. We need to recover a deeper sense of the whole range of relationships which have no sexual overtones. Here is a large area for future moral exploration.

Ambivalence towards risk

Finally, a word on the notion of "safe sex'. This is the slogan which lies at the heart of the government's programme: there can be "safe sex" if you use a condom. I am willing to accept it as an interim slogan. But what it ignores—and this will become increasingly apparent in the long run—is the fact that part of the attraction of sex lies in the element of risk. At its best, as I have already pointed out, sex involves a kind of vulnerability; and if this cannot be the deep personal vulnerability which I have been commending, then it shows itself in other ways. Isn't it the case that there are many deliberate failures to use contraceptives, in what might otherwise be compromising circumstances, because the risk involved in not using them is part of the excitement— and indeed, for some people, the only sort of context which makes sexual relations possible?

There are those who are best stimulated sexually by illicit adventures, and the search for this kind of titillation is now a particularly dangerous and destructive part of our culture. Linked with this is the ambivalence of our society towards risks in general. We worry enormously about some very small risks, yet in other contexts we commend and encourage people for taking risks. Dangerous sports are an obvious example. The more absurd and risky the things people do, the more likely they are to be treated as heroes. We have to face the paradox that "safe sex" is not likely to appeal to the more adventurous and highly regarded members of the population, because unsafe sex is seen as an assertion of manhood. The "macho image" in young men is particularly strong.

Thus we not only need to shift our perception of what intimacy entails; we also need to shift our perception of adventurousness. Perhaps they can be shifted together by suggesting that promiscuity is in the end a cop-out, an escape, a way of getting cheap thrills through flouting conventions, even though the conventions are now fairly weak. What promiscuity *avoids* is precisely that adventurous self-giving which lies at the heart of true intimate relationships. The excitement of sex ought to be the excitement of knowing another person at that deep level, including the risk of accepting the responsibility of children. I believe that one of the things our society desperately needs to recover is this kind of understanding of personal relationships.

A last Christian comment. Unfortunately the Churches have a disastrous reputation for simply laying down laws about sex, while ignoring the fact that such laws frequently act as an invitation to revolt. I believe we need to concentrate more on the good news; and the good news is that human beings have within themselves the possibilities of entering into these deep and lasting relationships, that by the grace of God we have the possibility of faithfulness, that we can accept and work through our vulnerability and with God's help make something good out of it. I hope the message most loudly heard from the Churches is in the end a message of faith and hope and love, and an assurance of personal worth. These are the qualities most desperately needed if we are to face together this terrible scourge.

23 | Privilege and responsibility

Donald English
General Secretary of the Methodist Home Mission Division

The Church will make its best contribution to the problem created by Aids if it remembers what it means to be the Church. It is fatally easy for Christians, in the best interests of relating to secular society, to forget that we have a distinctive viewpoint to offer.

The Church is concerned with truth. At the heart of this concern is the conviction that the being and purposes of God determine what truth is. If part of that truth is that dangerous behaviour brings disaster then the Church must say so. It is no part of compassion to gloss over the cause of suffering. Compassion for all the world's population requires clarity about the major ways in which Aids has spread so far through sexual promiscuity, both heterosexual and homosexual. It gives us no pleasure to point it out, nor is a judgmental spirit appropriate as one points out that sad fact. But it is true and needs to be stated.

The Free Church tradition lays great stress on the importance of the Bible as the basis for faith. The doctrine of Creation as taught in scripture emphasises the privilege of humanity (made in the image of God) and the responsibility of humanity (to walk in harmony with God). Once the privilege is taken as a right, to be used against God's will (portrayed in Genesis 3 in terms of the wilful eating of the apple of the tree of life), then the harmony is broken, with dire consequences (expulsion from the garden in the Genesis 3 story). This is a rhythm of life on earth. When we seek to grasp what we have as a gift, and use it to our own ends contrary to God's purposes, first disorder then disaster results.

The double tragedy takes us still further. Human responsibility in biblical terms is not limited to our relationship to God. We are also responsible to and for one another. As we come to birth, survive and grow through the care and concern of others, so also we can be deeply harmed by, and can deeply harm others. None of us can live for himself or herself alone.

This is the case with so human an experience as sexual relationship. God's purpose is expressed in the Bible that sexual

154

intercourse is intended for the secure intimacies of a loving relationship within marriage. Once we move outside that relationship and into casual sex, then we are in danger of using sex purely for our enjoyment; and still worse of using other people as objects for our gratification, not persons needing to be loved. The result in hurt people and debased human relationships is often too evident. Venereal disease has been one price paid for prostituting a lovely gift of God. The rapid spread of Aids is another.

The defence of minorities

Concern for truth works both ways, however. The Church must be equally clear about the origin of the disease and about the fact that it was not caused either by homosexual or illicit heterosexual behaviour. Christians will support plans for extensive research in this area. In the strictest sense all the sufferers are victims of a disease for whose origin they are not responsible.

Another strong Free Church tradition has been the defence and development of minorities in society, whether religious or political, who are in danger of being persecuted or neglected. Part of the reason is that Free Church men or women members were persecuted minorities in earlier centuries. We have fought for our own right to worship according to conscience, to receive education in each of the institutions available to others. For the same reason Free Church people, particularly Methodists, were prominent in the beginning of the trade union movement.

The hard question now is whether the Free Church passion to support small persecuted groups can extend to Aids sufferers. There is a great danger of accurately identifying the spread of Aids with sexual promiscuity and drug abuse and then drawing the conclusion that they should be left to suffer what they have brought upon themselves. Mercifully (literally) this is not the biblical tradition. Jesus showed particular compassion for the outcasts. It is significant that it should be shepherds who heard news of his birth, since they were by their profession religious outcasts. Again and again he was found offering care and compassion where no "decent" person would go. If persecuted groups are defensible by right, and if the sick are worthy of God's love and care, the Christian will be in the foreground of caring for Aids sufferers, supporting and staffing hospices for their treatment, and protecting them from persecution.

I believe that, from time to time, groups as large as nations have an opportunity for a decisive change in direction. The ingredients of such an opportunity are first an issue serious enough to be a challenge to everyone, second a process whereby everyone has the necessary information to decide on a change; and third, the appropriate leadership which points in the right way.

Faced by a challenge to the freedom of Europe in the late 1930's, the British people had to make a choice about how much their freedom mattered. In my judgment a right choice was made, horrific though the consequences were. Not many years later a prime minister told us we "had never had it so good". We ignored the other things he told us, and then made the wrong choice. We launched ourselves on a course of possessing more and more while making less and less, a course of self-indulgence for which we are still paying the price. We have another such choice now. It is a choice about how we treat other people, not least other people's bodies. This decision is not an isolated matter, although its link with Aids may give that impression. It is in fact part and parcel with all our other decisions about how we treat other people across barriers of distinction, male and female, rich and poor, black and white, old and young, north and south. Selfishness in one relationship makes selfishness in another one that much easier.

Since Free Church Christians have traditionally sought to call the nation to reflect on its Christian origins and duties it is high time now, together with all those who care about such things to raise a cry for compassion and justice in our treatment of one another, and to set the example. The emergence of Aids in our culture provides just such a moment. The seriousness of the situation can hardly be exaggerated. The figures for deaths in this country alone underline that. The information is being disseminated widely. The government is seeking to make the choices plain from the standpoint of prudence. The Church must offer leadership in terms of what is morally true.

There is a third point about truth. It requires careful judgment. However much the Church wishes people—and especially young people—to adopt disciplined relationships, it should not do so by following the policy of stimulating craven fear in our population. Our young people are already subjected to too much external pressure which exploits them. To frighten people may momentarily cause more restraint, but it is no basis for a sustained change of lifestyle. For that, careful, balanced decisions are required including those by people who influence our standards in society. To inform people of the consequences of certain actions in a way which causes them to give up such actions is one thing: to exploit them by causing terror will in the end be counter-productive. It could also lead to scapegoating and even to attacks on communities blamed for the epidemic. Already there is evidence of attacks on homes and groups, and on individuals in the street. Christians will wish to do nothing which remotely encourages such outrages. What is worse, under such pressures sex becomes a subject associated either with fear on the one hand, or a calculated risk of one's own, or someone else's life on the other, thus losing much of its beauty and meaning.

Emptying death of its threat

From beginning to end the true Christian insight about life depends upon a grateful receiving of God's gifts, like sex, and of using such gifts in a spirit of true love, love of God and love of others. One of the most memorable words in the New Testament is the single sentence, "perfect love casts out fear". There is much more lasting good from such sentiments than from an approach which frightens.

There is another reason why Christians cannot be satisfied with a policy based on fear. It gives the impression that death is the worst thing that can happen to us. Christians don't believe that. At the heart of the Christian faith is the death and resurrection of Jesus Christ. Our sacraments and our preaching declare that people can share Christ's dying and rising in a way which empties death of its threat. This central Christian tenet of faith and experience means that we do have something very deep indeed to offer to sufferers. The evidence from hospices for those dying of diseases like cancer and Aids enables us to speak even of hope and peace in such circumstances. This, as well as sheer human need, is the inspiration of our care and compassion for Aids sufferers, which will take many forms—from care for relatives and friends to participation in the development of hospices. The decision of the Mildmay Hospital to open a ward for Aids sufferers is surely a move to be welcomed by us all. They will need great support financially. This is one sign of a positive Christian response.

There is another point of deep significance here. Christian compassion for those who suffer and die from Aids, as for those who suffer or die from any other distressing disease, is based on our Lord's experience on the cross. His Cry of Dereliction means that God does understand and identify with our lowest moments of depression and despair. His Cry of Triumph means that the low point need not be the end. The threat of Aids raises again the question of how relevant the Christian gospel is to the modern world. Out of the heart of our message there is a place where deep can speak to deep. We are privileged humbly to make that clear.

Against this background the Christian advocacy of marriage as the proper setting for sexual relationships is not a matter of simply retaining part of the standards (though that is an honoured part of the tradition). It is rather to affirm the reality of enrichment through life-long married partnerships. It also has to do with the nature of God, and of his world. It is about achieving harmony with the business of being properly alive.

24 | Only a moral revolution can contain this scourge

Immanuel Jakobowits
Chief Rabbi

I have delayed publicly expressing a view on the awesome menace of Aids now hanging like a monstrous medieval plague over mankind, despite pressures from within my community and beyond to make some authentic Jewish pronouncement. This is due not merely to the fact that most authoritative Jewish statements on the moral issues were made thousands of years ago.

The earliest sources of Jewish law and morality are quite unambiguous. The Bible brands homosexual relationships as a capital offence (Lev 20.13), and execrates any sexual licentiousness as an abomination, whether in the form of premarital "harlotry" (Deut 23.18) or of extramarital adultery (Lev 20.10). Equally stern are the warnings of national doom consequent on any defiance of these principles: the land itself will "vomit out" peoples violating these injunctions (Lev 18.28–29).

My hesitation in adding a Jewish voice to the many religious and moral statements already widely publicised, and worthy of endorsement, has been accentuated by the uncompromising nature of these biblical strictures. The difficulties go beyond the dilemma of choosing between soothing platitudes and unpalatable truths.

I am still racked by doubts on how to react to such a horrendous threat, how to address an age not exactly attuned to the puritan language of the Bible, how to transcend the perplexities which baffle medical and government experts, and how to present deeply held convictions without causing offence, panic, or disdain for the very teachings I espouse.

Questions with no easy answers

There are questions to which I simply know of no categorical answers. Some are practical: is it right to advocate "safe sex"? Or, should all citizens be subjected to screening tests to identify carriers and, if so, how is this information to be used? Some questions are theological: can a disease like this, patently discriminating against some sections of society, be attributed to divine wrath, or altogether be judged in moral terms?

And some are purely human: how can one reassure without spreading complacency, warn without condescension or self-righteousness and highlight the horrific without inducing immunity to shock by horror? Altogether, are habits and behaviour susceptible to change by moral exhortation, by publicity campaigns, or even by medical information? Inscrutable as the answers may as yet be, and rudimentary as may be our understanding of the long-term effects of Aids and its spread, not to mention the prospects of halting its ravages, certain facts seem incontrovertible as a basis for some conclusions in the light of Jewish insights and moral principles.

Both at the individual and the public level, we are certainly never entitled to declare a particular form of suffering as a punishment for a particular manifestation of wrongdoing. We can no more divine why some people endure terrible ills without any apparent cause than we can comprehend why others prosper although they clearly do not deserve their good fortune.

Even less are we justified in being selective, subjecting some scourges to this moral analysis while exempting others (Aids, yes; but earthquakes or floods or droughts, no). There is no such simplistic relationship between evil and misfortune, if only because there are too many exceptions. According to Jewish exegesis, the prophet Isaiah had his lips scorched because

159

he sinned in saying, "I dwell in the midst of a people with unclean lips" (Is 6.5–6).

The inevitable price we pay

There is all the difference—even if the distinction is a fine one—between ascribing massive suffering to personal or social depravity as a divine visitation, and warning that such depravity may *lead* to terrible consequences. If I warn a child not to play with fire, and it ignores the warning and gets burned, the hurt is not a punishment but simply a consequence. If people recklessly indulge in infidelity and end up in the agony of a broken marriage, they suffer no vengeance; they simply pay the inevitable price for moral negligence or turpitude.

Public information campaigns should therefore be explicit and unequivocal: Aids is the price we pay for the "benefits" of the permissive society which, helped by the pill, liberal legislation and more enlightened attitudes, has demolished the last defences of sexual restraint and discipline, leading to a collapse of nature's self-defence against degeneracy.

An even greater price in human misery than deaths from Aids is being paid for violating the imperatives of sexual morality: the devastation of the family, with millions of casualties, especially among young people driven to vice and crime by the absence of a loving home.

The provision of condoms, condoning and facilitating sexual irresponsibility, is therefore hardly the answer, even if they temporarily reduce the transmission of Aids. They would only increase the ravages of personal degradation and social disintegration. In any case, what has to be carefully weighed is individual safety against the erosion of public standards. The principle is illuminated by a striking precedent—Jewish law and thought must invariably search for guidance in earlier sources.

A leading 15th-century Spanish-Jewish scholar objected to the establishment of facilities for communally controlled prostitution to keep licentiousness from running wild—even if this objection meant failing to prevent married partners from committing the capital offence of adultery (as implied in the Ten Commandments, Judaism makes no difference between killing a person and killing a marriage). He argued that however culpable individual indiscipline is, its mitigation cannot be sanctioned at the expense of the slightest public compromise with the Divine Law.

160

True, in Jewish law the saving of life overrides all religious precepts. But even this pro-life stance has three cardinal exceptions: forbidden liaisons, murder and idolatry are proscribed even at the cost of life. This, too, would seem to rule out recourse to any measures, such as condoms for unmarrieds, which would encourage indecent conduct, though the rule might be invoked to treat more leniently the distribution of clean needles for drug-abusers.

No less important than clean needles are clean speech, clean thoughts and clean conduct. What will be crucial is the cultivation of new attitudes calculated to restore reverence for the generation of life and the enjoyment of sexual pleasure exclusively within marriage. Nothing short of a moral revolution will in time contain the scourge. The role of governments in achieving these objectives is admittedly limited. Morality cannot be legislated, nor can politicians and civil servants become preachers. But the administrators of our national affairs cannot remain morally neutral either, when the eventual cost may be counted in millions of lives.

Governments can help to refine human behaviour—for instance, by opposing any legislation liable to weaken the bonds between husband and wife or parents and children. Equally, governments can, by the careful use of language in official speech and documents, eliminate from the common vocabulary the kind of euphemisms or misnomers that make perversions acceptable. I think of words like "gay" for homosexual, "heterosexual" for normal, "safe sex" for inadmissable indulgence, and "stable relationships" for unmarried couples.

The Jewish experience demonstrates that in the final analysis only spiritual power is invincible as a shield against lust. This is perhaps reflected in observant Jews, however addicted to smoking, finding the Sabbath prohibition against lighting a cigarette far more effective than the most alarming health warnings in securing complete abstention from smoking for one day in seven.

They have also discovered that a conscience so trained prevails even in the most intimate relations between husband and wife. The religious ban on any physical contact for some 12 days in every normal month, regularly rejuvenating the marriage through an iron self-discipline, achieves more than the most skilled marriage counsellor could in regulating the rhythm of love and longing. Natural urges can be bridled in submission to a higher law.

161

What is needed, then, is a massive campaign mobilising government resources and citizens of all faiths and of none to strive for moral excellence, to avoid the arousal of passions in literature and entertainment, to extol the virtues of fidelity, and to promote the utmost compassion for those struck by a hideous killer as a result of failings which may not be theirs but the society's into which they were born, and which to ennoble is the charge of us all.

Every action to promote these ideals has now become a lifesaving operation—including saving marriages as the sole legitimate origin of all human life.

25 | Longing for tenderness

Benedict Ramsden

Diocesan preacher to the Russian Orthodox Church in Britain

The primary pastoral ministry is the proclamation of the good news of salvation. Faced with Aids, the Church has first of all the duty and the ability to announce that faith, hope and love are still possible. Her speaking of faith should be above question. Her message of hope should be of such an authority that no-one can confuse it with propaganda put about to allay public panic. Above all, her ministries of loving must not be mistakable for a fringe activity in the voluntary sector of caring. They must speak, wordlessly perhaps but with especial power, of the love that is able to cast out fear.

Fear is in the air. This is no new thing. My own generation has lived most of its life in the shadow of two global fears. Most of us have arrived at some sort of accommodation with those fears but I suspect this has more to do with habit than with Christian hope. The Church is now faced with a challenge. Future generations will judge her by her response. It would be tragic if they were to look back on us as we do on the Church under Hitler, which seems to be credited with little more than noticing that the trains were running on time. Such failures are not simply blots on the Church's copybook. They profoundly undermine the world's expectations of her.

In my experience, so far as Aids is concerned, these expectations are not very high and little seems to be happening to raise them. I have heard from several Christian quarters that Aids is a divine visitation upon the permissive society; a blessing that will restore Christian marriage and morality to the public sector. In so far as anyone has sought my advice, it has largely been about the dangers of catching Aids from the chalice. A very few Christians have spoken to me of the special ministry to the dying that will be needed. Living as I do with people who tend to be pushed to the fringes of the community, I have already been faced with the question of domestic contact with those who may be HIV-positive and have thus had a small glimpse of the needs and fears involved.

First of all, I do not believe in a God of selective vindictiveness; nor in one whose aim is so bad that in clobbering the permissive society he hits those who need blood transfusions as well. Mine is a good God who loves mankind. He has created humanity, not for destruction but for communion with himself. He has, from the time of Noah (to whom he promised never again to destroy mankind), covenanted his mercy to mankind. In Christ he has identified himself totally with us, working out our salvation by an act that brought the ultimate good out of human wickedness. This is the ground of Christian hope and courage. It is not a vague optimism nor any guarantee that I shall spend the whole of my lifetime in cosy comfort and complacency, but a basis for special kind of living, epitomised by the Martyrs, from which despair is excluded.

Supporting celibacy

One response to the present situation has been the recommendation of changes in sexual habits. There are some indications that this advice is being heeded. It may be that terror is inspiring a move towards a sexual ethic which, if it were inspired by love, might be called Christian. Even if this new lifestyle is only a parody of the chastity toward which the Church exhorts her children, it would seem that we have a pastoral need — the support of the celibate — in which the Church should by now have nearly two thousand years of experience. This new situation of reluctant mass celibacy is an opportunity for exercise of that experience.

163

It is well known to monastic teachers that those embracing the celibate life need a great deal of loving support, both from their communities in general and from their spiritual fathers in particular. Chastity is not easy and lonely chastity is even harder. The Church has not always been either successful or sympathetic in her ministry to human sexuality. Perhaps now that Mr and Ms Average are trying to live in a way that resembles the Christian paradigm, they may have more hope of finding some claim upon the tenderness of the Christian community. Most human beings, men as well as women, have a more desperate and aching need of tenderness than they have of sex. It is within the experience of tenderness that they are likely to grow to a sexuality, celibate or otherwise, that is worthy of them.

The experience of touch

Both in her solemn liturgy and in the informalities that her children share between themselves, the Orthodox Church shows a particular tenderness. This tenderness is not an accident of ethnic custom but a realisation of the Incarnation and the consequent sacredness of the human body. Gestures of touching, embracing, and kissing; the exquisitely tender sacramental signs of anointing, the familiar sight of the confessor with his arm around the penitent, the solemn ministries and dignities afforded to the body and the senses; all bear witness to that divine tender-love of mankind of which the liturgy so often speaks. To a new and growing number of people, these things will have a special significance.

It is likely that Aids sufferers will find themselves not only longing for tenderness but wanting for any kind of human contact at all. There is a growing climate of fear. People speak of a new plague. There is added to all the other terrors of the victim, the ultimate horror of isolation. In such a context, the Orthodox experience of touch is not merely moving and beautiful, it is a proclamation of peace and hope, a sort of silent gospel.

On the morning on which I write these words, the media are full of a visit by the Princess of Wales to an Aids ward. The thing emphasised above all else is that she shook hands without gloves with a series of Aids patients. If such a gesture is of so much significance, it behoves the Orthodox to make sure that they do not use their traditional tenderness simply as the characteristic behaviour of an "in" group. Like all the activities

164

of the Church, they are either ministries of Christ or they are worse than nothing.

A ministry to fear

One should need to say little of the Church's ministry to the dying. She is uniquely able in this area. One has only to see the impact made upon the world by Mother Teresa to see that the secular world is powerfully moved when this ministry is fully lived. The Church must not only administer consolation but must speak out, as she especially can, about the possibility of meaning, beauty and dignity in death. As in Calcutta, the new situation is particularly poignant in that it is largely the young who are dying or living in the certain expectation of death— and as the situation goes on there is more and more danger of their dying alone.

There is already a need of a special ministry to fear. Fear is not allayed by propaganda. The greatest assurance to the fearful is the presence of those who are unafraid. In this situation the Church's handling of such questions as the safety of the ministration of the chalice becomes a matter of significance. Some practical expedients have already been adopted in parts of America which seem to me to run the risk of increasing fear by pandering to it. Fear must never supplant reverence for and faith in the reality of the sacrament. There is a need of a sensitivity to, and an allaying of, the fears of a frightened laity in a way that leaves the power and dignity of the sacrament intact.

I regret somewhat the introduction of any distinction between lay and clerical ministries in this matter since witness to the gospel in love and fearlessness is the common vocation of all. There is, however, in the finishing of the Holy Gifts after communion, a special call on the heroism of the priest or deacon. The Church has always asked of the priest a particular kind of heroism in witnessing to the gospel in its fulness. Orthodoxy does not for example make concessions in the matter of divorce to the clergy, as it does to the laity. Perhaps then the priest has a particular opportunity to show that absence of fear which is a mark of love. His role in relation to the Divine Gifts should always be a witness to his faith that the sacrament of Christ's Body and Blood is not a means for the proliferation of infection but for the healing of soul and body and for immortal life.

26 | To serve rather than preach

Gerald Priestland

Writer and broadcaster on religious affairs and former
foreign correspondent of the BBC

No spokesperson, no committee even, can lay down the Quaker
law on Aids. Being anti-authoritarian from the beginning, the
Society of Friends dislikes issuing codified guidance on the
burning issues of the day. This may seem curious for an
organisation which has long lived up to its neck in practical
concerns like penal reform, mental health, refugee relief and
peace, but one would like to think it reflects the Quaker view
that while faith should be expressed in action rather than
argument, guidance is always available by waiting upon the Holy
Spirit "after the manner of Friends". That is to say, in unambitious
but attentive contemplation in the context of the world, rather
than by trying to wrestle the world's problems into the context of
yesterday's doctrines and scriptural interpretations.

Sophisticated theologians will at once sniff the danger of
trendy antinomianism. That danger has always haunted
Quakers from the earliest times when they had to disengage
themselves from the libertinism of the Ranters. But they did so,
successfully, largely through a rigorous system of consensus-
forming. We may not have dogma, but we certainly have
tradition, and on the ethical side it still includes a strong element
of puritanism. There are not many people who regard Quakers
as notorious underminers of old-fashioned family values. In
Britain, anyway, most of us are too old for that.

We no longer disown our children for marrying outside the
Society, but we have our legally recognised form of marriage
which we refer to as a "lifelong comradeship". The closest we
have come to defining a philosophy of sexual relationship is in
the following passage from our *Advices* to members:

> Throughout life, rejoice in the power and beauty of those
> friendships which grow in depth, understanding and mutual
> respect. At all times love and value "that of God" in your
> friend. No relationship can be a right one which makes use of
> another person through selfish desire.

166

It will be noticed that this passage makes no distinction as to sex. Although the *Advices* are currently under revision, it is this writer's impression that most Friends would prefer to leave it this way rather than make it explicitly applicable to homosexual or heterosexual (or indeed platonic) relationships. Among some Australian and American Quakers there have been loud demands to write in the gays and even to provide some kind of formal wedding for them. This had led to scandal and threats of schism. Perhaps it is typical of English Friends—who tend to be quietly liberal but modest and tactful—that they would prefer privacy to be both granted and observed in such matters. Some may call this hypocrisy: others good manners.

Hostility to the notion of a judgmental God

This is not to say that British Quakers pretend that gay people are invisible. There is a recognised homosexual group within the Society and many gays seem to feel comfortable in the nonjudgmental atmosphere of a Quaker Meeting for Worship. Some readers will recall the uproar caused by the publication in 1963 of the pamphlet "Towards a Quaker View of Sex", produced by a working party of psychologists, teachers and lawyers, which helped to prepare the ground for the eventual decriminalisation of private adult homosexual behaviour. By no means all Quakers approved of it. To some extent it has been overtaken by events—notably the appearance of Aids—but along with other factors it undoubtedly helped to influence Friends in a non-condemnatory direction.

There is an optimism about human nature at the heart of English Quakerism. The Evangelical streak has mostly washed out of us and we are not much interested—perhaps we are too little interested—in sin. Our long experience of the penal system has made us positively hostile to the notion of punishment. We have also been much occupied with the sciences. All of this has combined to make Friends averse to any view of Aids as a judgment of God upon an immoral generation which has flouted his law and wallowed in its own lusts. It is a judgment only in the sense that the biblical rules are biologically sound and that to ignore them is to invite the natural consequences.

Drawing upon the Quaker tradition the present writer cannot believe that we have a cruelly indiscriminate God punishing not just the sodomite, the promiscuous and the junkie but the innocent haemophiliac, the infected wife and the babe in her

167

womb. God is not thundering "Serve them all right!" but weeping "Why wouldn't they listen to me!" Aids may be a consequence of the moral confusion of the permissive generation, but only in part—why did it originate in the first place? Anyone who believes it to be an awarded punishment must believe that the Black Death, the Great Plague, smallpox and syphilis were punishments in their day—but for what great sins? And they were not effective in reforming mankind. A God who tried that method again could not have learned very much, could hardly be a God of Love.

It is many generations since Quakers saw any point in stalking the country lecturing and threatening people on God's behalf. Our purpose now is to worship him and serve his people in his honour. Just as Christ did not hesitate to touch the leper and was not restrained by the sins of the sick he healed, nor should we be. We are told that we shall be judged according to how we cared for the unfortunate: we shall not be excused for drawing back from those we disapprove of. Thus service to those dying of Aids stands as a test of our devotion to Christ which we dare not fail, however lofty our personal morals.

Remembering the Third World

We in the West can be confident that, in time, science will find a cure. This will be difficult—there will be setbacks—but the record of science is good and the resources are there if we will them to come forward. At the same time Aids is a warning that disease can always keep a jump ahead of us, that death itself cannot be abolished. In any case the sufferings of our comfortable world, however dreadful by our standards, will be as nothing compared with what is inexorably happening in the Third World, especially Africa. We shall not be forgiven if we become so absorbed in pity and pride for ourselves that we turn our backs upon that helpless and vulnerable continent which we shall have to succour without judgment or sense of superiority.

Some good Christians already find the official Aids campaign in Britain shocking. Catholics especially deplore its mechanical attitude towards "safe sex". Where is there a word about saying no, about virginity, chastity, fidelity? Hardly anywhere, and perhaps that is a measure of the general loss of confidence in Christian teaching. That being so, it is hardly for the State to take over that business. Aids is now a matter of public safety and the State has to tackle it as practically as it can. There is nothing to stop the Church preaching and putting up posters for any who will heed them. But when the train has lost its brakes, we have to find ways of stopping it—not just deplore the lack of proper maintenance work in the past.

Some sternly biblical pastors would like to drive homosexuals out of the Church altogether, or at least humiliate them, though they are the people who need its understanding, even where its blessing is hardly possible, more than anyone. In a world where the Gospel comes too late, what purpose do such gestures serve other than to wash the hands of the self-righteous? And what service is that to God?

Quakers—of whom there are barely 20,000 in Great Britain and Ireland—may be criticised for having spread their sympathies too thin in too many directions. They have few resources to spare now for an effective contribution against Aids, and must envy the Catholic Church in particular for its pioneering in the hospice movement—a place where Friends would willingly have been if they had not been elsewhere. If it is the duty of a Church to teach people how to live, we would rather do that by living than by talking. And if our brothers and sisters are suffering, we would rather serve them than preach at them.

PART VII | The Christian and the secular

27 | The flaws in the government response

David Alton

Member of Parliament for Liverpool, Mossley Hill, and Liberal chief whip

Even if the most lurid and scaremongering headlines are ignored, the only certainty about Aids is that it is potentially the greatest threat to health worldwide this century. The statistics are frightening. Aids is the biggest single killer of men in their 30s in New York; in parts of Africa whole communities are infected with the Aids virus; and countries like Zambia may be economically and socially destroyed. In Britain, the figures for those with full-blown Aids are still low, but the Department of Health and Social Security expects 4,000 deaths by the end of 1989.

The first question when considering the government response to Aids is to ask how swiftly they have reacted to the crisis. While the government has achieved much which has been constructive and deserves the praise and support of all the political parties, I believe that by failing to take the initiative back in 1983-4 it stored up problems for itself and has moved disastrously slowly on several important measures. In examining these achievements, the background to them, and the pressures that have constrained the government it is worth commenting on what could have been done and what must still be done.

Refusal to recognise the problem of Aids

The response to Aids, whether in or out of Parliament, has been influenced by ignorance, caused partly—and naturally—by the nature of the disease. It was not until 1983 that the causative virus was identified and while a vast amount has been learnt in a very short time, a great deal has still to be discovered, not least a cure or vaccine. This lack of knowledge was exacerbated by our western view of the world, which led to the African situation going largely unnoticed. Aids, as a result, became associated with homosexuality as the first cases appeared in American homosexuals.

173

The "gay plague" label which followed has had several serious consequences, internationally and domestically. A number of countries, which do not recognise the existence of homosexuality, also refused to recognise the existence of Aids, thus losing valuable time and research experience for themselves and the rest of the world. In Britain, intolerance of minorities has been compounded by fear of Aids and has led to additional stress and suffering for those already afraid that they might be at risk. Most serious of all, the government has had to try and correct the indifference among many heterosexuals. If the government had acted back in 1983, the extent of Aids in the homosexual population would have been less and it would have spread slower in the heterosexual population. Much suffering might have been spared.

The government finally launched its advertising campaign in late 1986, but only after a year of pressure from medical experts. It was notable that the campaign was aimed first, both in the newspapers and subsequently on television, at explaining that Aids could affect anyone. The government slogan was "Don't die of ignorance", but the disease's long incubation period—up to five years or more—ensured that for a number of both homosexuals and heterosexuals the slogan was simply too late. Even so, the message still needs to be accepted not least in Parliament itself that Aids is not caused or spread simply through a person's sexuality. Certain sexual acts and lifestyles are a factor, and some heterosexuals are at much greater risk than many homosexuals. Hence the need for the advertising campaign to be blunt and explicit to ensure that the facts are understood.

Acting in the best interests of the community

As an MP who is a Catholic I appreciate that getting the facts across in the necessary blunt manner poses great problems for the government. Questions of sex bring with them questions of morality, not least for a government that would pride itself on supporting family values. Many Conservatives, in Parliament and outside, would rather wash their hands of the situation and reject effective measures either because they believe that people with Aids are being punished for a lifestyle which offends God or because measures to control the spread of Aids also offend against religious teaching. The then Scottish health minister, John McKay, asserted that Aids was a totally self-inflicted

174

disease and, effectively, that victims should blame themselves. Another Tory MP complained that the advertising campaign, at first nothing like as strong as medical advisers wished, was brutal.

No political party can or should ignore the views of the many people who for religious or other reasons advocate a moral approach to life, and who believe in chastity without marriage and monogamy within. The Churches, while remembering the value of Christian compassion, clearly have an important view to put. However, it is up to each and every one of us, guided by our Church or convictions, to choose our manner of behaviour. No government can forget that it acts for all the people and that in our multicultural society a government-imposed morality is both impractical and wrong. The government must ensure that it acts in the best interests of the whole community even if this means offending parts of it. It must also ensure that individuals are fully aware of the consequences of their actions both for themselves and for the community. I believe, for these reasons, that the balanced message of stressing the need for one partner while promoting safer sex if this is impossible is the right one.

In a debate on Gavin Strang's Bill to Control the Spread of Aids, a Tory MP asked why all the effort on a largely self-inflicted disease, when there were many suffering from other diseases who needed support. His view was in a minority even if everyone also wished that more were done for health generally. The nature of Aids increases the pressure on the government. People with Aids need acute care, sometimes in hospital, at other times in the community. Yet the number of acute hospital beds has been consistently cut over the past few years and, even if prejudice can be overcome, community care is still a concept rather than a reality. Too often it is a case of dumping, rather than caring, in the community.

The health service simply does not have the beds, facilities or staff to cope with the numbers of Aids patients. The Department of Health and Social Security disclosed to my colleague, Archy Kirkwood MP, that the cost of treating an Aids patient was between £10,000 and £20,000. Despite encouraging news on recent Aids research, a cure or vaccine must be at least five years away. It is thus no wonder that the view that people with Aids should be left to die was a minority one even within the Conservative party.

Greater resources needed

The government took a number of early measures which were sensible and uncontroversial. An expert advisory committee was set up, complemented in 1986 by a special Cabinet committee chaired by Lord Whitelaw to coordinate measures across departments. Since 1982 Aids cases have been voluntarily reported to the Communicable Disease Surveillance Centre, as have figures on HIV-positive tests. Warnings to blood donors not to donate blood if they came from a high risk group were issued, and the very low and static numbers of positive results among blood donors show that this measure is working. Since the end of 1984, heat-treated Factor VIII has been available for haemophiliacs—although the country will not be fully self-sufficient in Factor VIII until mid-1987. Guidelines have been issued to health service staff, although they are not always followed, and to employers.

Other issues are more controversial and the government's record less praiseworthy. Many of the services designed to care and treat people with Aids demand expansion and greater resources. Urgently needed are greater hospital provision, especially in the four Thames regions; community care facilities and trained staff to enable patients to remain in their homes; hospice accommodation; sufficient provision for sexually transmitted disease clinics to meet the demand for testing and provide counsellors. Yet up to the end of 1985, when there were already 108 cases of Aids, only £2 million had been allocated for these areas and for research.

The figures for 1987–1988 are more impressive: £7 million for patient care, £12.5 million for health education, and £14.5 million for research for the next three years. Yet these funds remain inadequate. The answers to questions I tabled in Parliament recently revealed that the Public Health Laboratory Service on Merseyside, which does all the local testing for HIV, tested 1,735 people in the first three months of this year compared with 249 in the first quarter of 1986. Staff and funding, however, remained constant and I was shocked to see the cramped room in which the work is undertaken when I recently visited the unit.

Doctors predict that £20 million will have to be diverted from other budgets to cope this year alone, and Department of Health and Social Security figures show that in 1988 the cost of caring for Aids patients will be between £20 and £30 million. The South East Thames Regional Health Authority asked for £4 million for this year. They received £700,000, yet £850,000 is needed to pay for heat-treated Factor VIII for haemophiliacs alone. Government staffing guidelines for hospitals ensure that medical staff at all levels are working under great pressure, and the bulk of the work is being done by academic rather than health service staff. The implications for the amount of time left for teaching and research are serious. Health authorities outside London are to receive no extra funding, yet they need resources now to enable them to plan for the future. In 1986 the independent College of Health estimated that at least £60 million per year was needed, figures that both the Alliance and the Labour Party have broadly accepted.

Norman Fowler came back from his visit to San Francisco and Amsterdam advocating the importance of caring for Aids patients within the community. The experience there shows that patients respond better in sympathetic surroundings and, anyway, it is a more civilised approach to people with Aids. Norman Fowler must back up his verbal support for community care with the needed resources, if only because the hospital beds are not going to be there.

Sharp dilemmas

The importance of continuing preventative measures must not be underestimated. The advertising campaign will be long-running, which is very welcome. The television companies deserve our congratulations for their imaginative contributions to raising the public awareness of Aids, which has partly made up for the sensationalist, unpleasant and often inaccurate coverage in the popular newspapers. More work is still needed, even if, we have seen, the government must tread warily. The dilemmas are also particularly sharp for the Roman Catholic Church as many of the advocated measures are against its teaching, but the Church of England too is under increasing pressure to take a more moralistic stance. Cardinal Hume has said, "We are dealing with an intrinsically moral question and not simply one of public health.... The Church wants to tackle promiscuity as the principal cause of infection". Edwina Currie MP has gone further by suggesting that "good Christians will not catch Aids".

The government, however, is being urged to provide free condoms, is promoting their use, and has sanctioned needle exchange systems for drug abusers in the major cities. On both issues the government message is double-edged: don't inject or sleep around, but take precautions if you must. I believe this is right. Aids means that many need to reevaluate their lifestyles. Yet the government does not have time to bring about changes in lifestyle, even if it were possible. The minister of health, Tony Newton, has said: "I disagree with the view that a moral crusade would be a sufficient answer to this problem". I believe that for this reason Alliance spokesmen have been right to advocate that condoms should be made more widely and freely available—not to encourage sex, certainly not to attack religious values, but because it may save lives in the future and may protect those who might otherwise not be in a position to protect themselves. While the government cannot ignore the moral question, they cannot afford to take a moral stance on behalf of people. They can only encourage people to make the right decisions for themselves.

The question of providing free syringes for drug addicts is at least as delicate as no-one wishes to encourage drug addiction. The alternative cannot be contemplated. In Edinburgh there are believed to be 3,000 HIV carriers linked to drug abuse and the problem is rapidly spreading to other cities. The problem is also rife on the Continent. One of the reasons for the rapid spread of HIV in Edinburgh appears to be that the police confiscated syringes, forcing addicts to share equipment. The low level of HIV in the drug community in Amsterdam shows the importance of special schemes to combat Aids. A similar scheme to provide help to addicts has been operating in Liverpool where excellent relationships between addicts and police have been built, and so the number of Aids cases is mercifully small. Methadone substitution and sympathetic counselling should be integral parts of any scheme. The delay in implementing such programmes in Britain is to be deeply regretted, but now that the government is finally tackling the problem, they deserve support.

The government's approach to research is deserving of rather less support. Research in all areas is admittedly paltry, but one might expect that the potential rewards to be derived from a cure or vaccine would justify the investment. Until this year, less than £.5 million was allocated for research. This has now been increased to £14.5 million over three years, although the principal researchers have repeatedly made requests for £10 million for the first year of spending. The method of allocation needs to be examined to ensure that funds reach the necessary recipients, who may not have time to comply with the present allocation rules.

178

Testing or screening for Aids poses a number of problems, not least the delay between infection and antibodies appearing in the blood, the lack of accuracy in the test itself, and the worrying fact that the virus appears to be mutating in, possibly, several forms. The government must plan ahead, and needs to be able to accurately estimate the possible number of cases. Voluntary testing, backed up by counselling, should be encouraged and back-up facilities must be provided on a scale commensurate with the problem.

Anonymous testing of blood samples routinely taken in hospital and screened for rubella and other diseases is another possibility. The government has rejected this at the moment because permission would not be sought for such testing and those found to be HIV-infected would not be informed. However, I believe that this is the least dangerous method of collecting general data and should be looked at again. The government has rejected, and must go on rejecting, compulsory mass screening, both for visitors to the country and the general population, and they have also rejected the possibility of isolating people with Aids. As they have said, both would be medically useless and socially deeply damaging.

The government has achieved much in many of the important areas, but increased resources have to be given now to enable health and local authorities to plan ahead and ensure that people with Aids are cared for in the best manner; for research for a cure and a vaccine; and to prevent the virus spreading any further. A national long term strategy is the best way to achieve this and should be strengthened by cross party talks to achieve a consensus and to give the government support to take the necessary measures.

For the Christian, a special responsibility exists. Diseases are not judgmental; although suffering, pain and the response which such a condition evokes in others can tell us a lot about them, ourselves, and our relationship with God. Jesus told us not to judge and he had special words of comfort for the sinner and sufferers alike. In St Matthews's gospel, Chapter 10, he puts a premium on hospitality and compassion. Anyone, he says, who turns his followers away will receive a fate worse than the citizens of Sodom and Gomorrah. That puts things into the right perspective and serves to remind us of how a Christian society should respond to the challenge which Aids provides.

28 | Aids, law and morals

Simon Lee

Lecturer in law at King's College, London

There is little to gain but much to lose through using the law in an attempt to solve the problems posed by Aids. Contrary to popular opinion, lawyers are the first to recognise the limits of law as an instrument of social change. Non-lawyers, however, have often had the Pavlovian response of seeking to change the law when faced with a moral, social or medical problem.

It is, therefore, an encouraging sign of the times that the government's response to this most devastating affliction of Aids has been to counter a modern plague by using modern techniques such as television or advertising. Even though there will be disagreements about the content of the advertising, by and large this method of education must be counted as an appropriate and constructive one, far better than unrealistically turning to the law for help.

The government advertising campaign has been asking us not to stand on our legal rights but to do something above and beyond what the law requires of us. We are legally entitled to be promiscuous but we are being asked to recognise that our legal rights are not what matters. We must not hide behind the law's minimal demands and forget our moral responsibilities. This is an important lesson for campaigners to learn. Of course, the law can have an educative role, but there are grave dangers in setting up law reform as the touchstone of society's response to a problem.

Blame for the permissive society

Thus, while it would give some people some satisfaction to pass a draconian law in response to Aids, we have to ask whether any law could help prevent the spread of Aids and, even if it could, whether it could only do so at an unacceptable cost to civil liberties. For example, at one extreme, some people might want to pass a law to incarcerate all Aids victims, all HIV carriers and all members of groups with an above average propensity to transmit the Aids virus. In the unlikely event that society could force such solitary confinement on a considerable proportion of citizens, should we do so given that it would involve the violation of those people's rights? The last time British law used such a severe method to counter sexually transmitted disease was a spectacular failure. The Contagious Diseases Acts 1866-69 provided for the compulsory detention, examination, isolation and treatment of women suspected of carrying venereal disease. Victorian values might have justified some action to counter the threat of VD but apparently these laws went too far for the Victorian public. Widespread unease with, and criticism of, the statutes soon led to their powers not being exercised and the laws were repealed in 1886.

One hundred years later, the law has moved even further away from that kind of approach to problems caused by sexual promiscuity. The Wolfenden Report in 1957, which examined the laws on prostitution and on homosexual practice, has sometimes been blamed for the permissive society which has in turn sometimes been blamed for Aids. Ten years later, the main recommendations of the report were passed onto the statute book by the Sexual Offences Act 1967.

But the report did not start from the premise that homosexual practice was a desirable moral option. It argued, on the contrary, that there were practical and civil libertarian reasons for the law to tolerate homosexual practice, notwithstanding its immorality. First, the law against homosexual practice was not working, it would be costly to enforce and it could only be enforced arbitrarily. Second, a decent society ought to respect people's privacy even if it disapproved of their lifestyle, unless and until that lifestyle threatened others.

Preventing harm to others

This traditional liberal view on when the law should intervene is most famously associated with John Stuart Mill, who wrote that "The only purpose for which power can be rightfully exercised over any member of a civilised community against his will is to prevent harm to others. His own good, either physical or moral, is not a sufficient warrant." But this phrase does not help us very much with Aids, or with much else.

As a general statement of the relationship between law and morality, the harm-to-others test begs all the important questions. "What is harm?" is precisely the problem with debates about, for example, pornography and surrogate motherhood. "Who are the others?" is precisely the problem with debates about, for instance, abortion and embryo experimentation.

However, it is clear that Aids *does* harm others. Nevertheless, that does not give society *carte blanche* in its reaction to the problem. Harm-to-others is a necessary but not a sufficient condition for intervention, according to Mill. Power *can* be rightfully exercised to prevent harm to others, says Mill. But he does not say that where harm-to-others is caused, we *must* use such power. Unfortunately, Mill does not give us more precise guidance as to when we should use society's power against the will of an individual. Presumably there remains a balancing exercise. We may have to decide whether intervention will be successful, calculate the harm caused by intervention and weigh it against the harm caused by the initial action.

Aids harms others, so we could pass laws to stop its transmission. But does homosexual activity in itself constitute "harm" for the purposes of Mill's approach? Aids has given a new twist to the old debate about decriminalising homosexuality. The Wolfenden Report in 1957 recommended the decriminalisation of homosexual acts between consenting adults in private. Its justification was "the importance which society and the law ought to give to individual freedom of choice and action in matters of private morality. Unless a deliberate attempt is to be made by society, acting through the agency of the law, to equate the sphere of crime with that of sin, there must remain a realm of private morality which is, in brief and crude terms, not the law's business."

Law cannot forbid all the vices

The Churches have sometimes given the impression that this approach is unacceptably permissive, yet there is great religious authority for accepting a distinction between law and morals. St Thomas Aquinas, for example, anticipated John Stuart Mill by some 600 years and Wolfenden by 700 years when he wrote that "Law is laid down for a great number of people of which the great majority have no high standard of morality, therefore it does not forbid all the vices from which upright men can keep away but only those grave ones which the average man can avoid and chiefly those which do harm to others and have to be stopped if human society is to be maintained, such as murder, theft and so forth." More recently, the Vatican Declaration on Abortion acknowledges the same point, in a phrase echoed in the recent Vatican statement on bioethics: "It is true that civil law cannot expect to cover the whole field of morality or to punish all faults. No-one expects it to do so. It must often tolerate what is in fact a lesser evil, in order to avoid a greater one." And the British archbishops' statement on abortion once again stresses that "we do not seek to have all Catholic moral teaching imposed by law".

Having emphasised that we need pastoral, social, moral and medical, rather than legal, responses to Aids, there are nevertheless at least four areas where we can see some legal problems arising from Aids. Yet in each case, I do not think that the law needs dramatic change and I do not think that the law can be a dramatic help.

The first issue is what the law should do if someone has sex without informing his partner that he is an Aids carrier? My immediate response is that a criminal punishment comes too late to help any infected partner. On the other hand, the law might possibly act as an additional deterrent and, in any event, there is a symbolic value in denouncing such callous behaviour. But this does not need a new law.

Crimes against the person

The most obvious charge where someone deliberately has unprotected sexual intercourse with another, concealing the fact that he or she is a HIV carrier, and where the partner subsequently dies, might seem to be murder or manslaughter. But there is a problem vis-à-vis Aids in that no murder or manslaughter charge will succeed if the death happens a year and a day after the act. This rule is rooted in the difficulties of earlier medical science in determining whether one particular blow "caused" a death which occurs a year or more later. This rule ought perhaps to be reconsidered in the light of medical advances in determining the cause of death and in the light of Aids, which will kill its victims over a much longer time span.

But the law has other criminal offences at its disposal. Other crimes against the person would be committed by the deliberate transmitter of Aids which could result in imprisonment for a considerable time. The Offences Against the Person Act 1861 is the relevant statute and section 23 is the most appropriate offence—maliciously administering any poison or other destructive and noxious thing so as thereby to endanger the life of such a person or to inflict upon him grievous bodily harm. There are difficulties in deciding whether the Aids micro-organism would come within the terms "poison or other destructive or noxious thing" but one suspects that judges would interpret the Act to include transmission of the Aids virus. So the Offences Against the Person Act 1861, especially when allied with the Criminal Attempts Act 1981, could act as a deterrent although I repeat my belief that anyone who is prepared to ignore their moral responsibilities is unlikely to be deterred by the threat of five years' imprisonment. Incidentally, although Aids is a new phenomenon, venereal disease has posed similar problems in relation to the criminal law.

The second issue is whether anyone who contracts Aids through the negligence of someone else, for example, by not checking a blood transfusion properly, can sue in the law of tort. Again, the answer is that they already could, depending on all the facts and depending on whether they could prove negligence according to the standards expected in the light of then current knowledge about Aids. So, again, no new law is needed. But again, compensation is not much consolation. Yet it is better than nothing and could help finance care.

The third problem is whether a doctor should breach confidence by informing the partners of Aids carriers. Once more, this is only a new variation on an old theme of doctors' dilemmas. Rights and duties sometimes conflict with other rights and duties. A doctor's duty to preserve confidentiality should not always prevail over his or her other moral and legal responsibilities. In this case, the doctor should obviously urge the patient to tell any partner of his condition. If the patient refuses to do so, the doctor might have to take the initiative for him. Of course, one must tread warily. To accuse someone falsely of Aids, for example, would open up to a defamation action. And widespread breaches of confidentiality might deter HIV carriers from approaching doctors, which could in turn put others at risk. But to fail to inform those who need to know by sheltering under an alleged absolute duty of confidentiality would itself be a mistake.

The fourth issue is whether high risk groups can use the law to protect themselves from discrimination or whether the law should countenance such discrimination. Drug addicts are already breaching the criminal law. The other high risk group, homosexuals, have two main fears regarding legal consequences—the possibility of a change in the criminal law on homosexual practice and the possibility of employment law failing to protect them from unfair dismissal.

Of course, those who argue that we should restore the old criminal law prohibitions on homosexual practice in response to Aids ought also, if they are to be consistent, argue for the criminalisation of adultery and all heterosexual promiscuity, since this too is a way of transmitting Aids. The fact that it is quite implausible that Parliament would criminalise hetero-sexual promiscuity, even in reaction to Aids, makes one suspect that the scourge of Aids is being used as an opportunity for law reform by those who have never accepted the Wolfenden-inspired liberalisation of the law on homosexual practice.

Law is a blunt instrument

However, I see no prospect of the Wolfenden-inspired Sexual Offences Act 1967, which decriminalised homosexual practice, being repealed or the old law restored. Such a law is unworkable, unenforceable and an undesirable invasion of privacy. This is not to command or even condone homosexual practice. It is rather to repeat the point that moral education, not legislation, should be the route for those who object to homosexual practice. The law is a technique, a tool of social control, which does some jobs well and some badly. Here there is disagreement on what the law should do and grave difficulties in the way of it doing anything constructive.

So far, all the legal responses to Aids which we have considered have focussed on efforts to stop the spread of Aids. Finally, let us turn to how the law might protect those suffering from Aids, those carrying the virus, or those whose lifestyle gives them a higher than average risk of catching Aids. These people are at risk of losing their jobs or of finding facilities, even medical care from their General Practitioners, denied to them. What can they do? I am afraid that the answer is much the same. Education of the wider community on problems and causes of Aids is the best protection for people with Aids against harassment and discrimination. The law is a blunt instrument, particularly when it comes to forcing employers, for example, to keep on the payroll a worker they would rather dismiss. Even before Aids, homosexuals have not been well protected by the law on unfair dismissal. In a Scottish case in 1980, for instance, a man lost his claim for unfair dismissal when he was sacked from a children's holiday camp simply because it was discovered that he was homosexual. The industrial tribunal thought that a "considerable proportion of employers would take the view that the employment of a homosexual should be restricted particularly when he is required to work in proximity to and contact with children". Even if homosexuals were better served by the law on unfair dismissal—which would require no change in the law but a change in the attitude of the industrial tribunals who interpret, and thus give content to, the legislation's broad guidelines of unfairness and unreasonableness—the law is usually satisfied by compensation for an unfair dismissal and rarely insists on reinstatement.

That illustrates the discrimination suffered even by those who do not have Aids and are not even HIV carriers. The problems multiply when we turn to consider these groups. Trevor Fishlock's "Letter from New York" in *The Times* of 5 September 1985, describes the kinds of discrimination faced by those actually suffering from Aids: "more than 4,300 people in this city have Aids, a third of all the cases in the United States, and New Yorkers are growing increasingly frightened as the fatal disease spreads . . . parents have won the support of New York's mayor in opposing the admission to school of children with Aids. Fear of the disease has been a significant factor. . . . Ever since Aids was first identified in the United States in June 1981, many of its victims have found themselves regarded with loathing. They have become the untouchables of the 1980s, thrown out of their homes and jobs and shunned by acquaintances. . .".

The journalist concludes with another city's legal response: "Los Angeles has passed a law to protect Aids victims from discrimination in housing, work and education. Homosexuals are concerned that the existence of the disease is increasing prejudice against them."

The United Kingdom is unlikely to follow Los Angeles' example. Whether or not we adopt a legal solution, however, the important point is that the New York approach of caving in to ignorance should be resisted. We should dispel fear of Aids victims and carriers rather than succumb to irrational prejudice. We should recognise the limitations of law rather than expect some magical remedy to emerge from Parliament in Westminster or the Royal Courts of Justice in the Strand. We should regard Aids as a moral and medical problem and look for a moral and medical solution without compromising the innocent but also without sacrificing our civil liberties.

APPENDIX

Many of the dioceses of England and Wales have taken action on Aids, including at the time of writing, Westminster, Arundel and Brighton, Birmingham, Brentwood, Cardiff, Liverpool, Portsmouth, Shrewsbury and Southwark. To find out more about the school guidelines, conferences or study days, ask your parish priest, who should know who in the diocese to contact to find out more.

"Aids: some guidelines for pastoral care" is a leaflet issued by the Church of England's Board for Social Responsibility (Church House Publishing, 60p).

An information and pastoral kit is available from the Aids and ARC programme of the Archdiocese of San Francisco. For further information write to Catholic Social Services, 50 Oak Street, San Francisco, Ca 94102, U.S.A.

"Housing Advice for People with Aids" from SHAC, 189a Old Brompton Road, London SW5 0AR.

"Facts about Aids for Drug Users", first 100 copies free from Standing Conference on Drug Abuse, 1-4 Hatton Place, Hatton Garden, London EC1N 8ND.

Aids helplines have been established in many towns and cities. The number can be found by calling directory enquiries. Some specific numbers are listed here:

Ireland

Confidential and free counselling service: CAIRE, 10 Fowndes Street, Dublin: 01-710895.

For drug abusers: Coolmine Therapeutic Community, 19 Lord Edward Street, Dublin 8: 01-782300.

Ana-Liffey Project, 13 Lower Abbey Street, Dublin 1: 01-786899.

Scotland

Scottish Aids Monitor, PO Box 169, Edinburgh EH1 3UU.

Edinburgh: 031-558 1167 (weekday evenings).
Dundee: 0343-25083 (office hours).
Glasgow: 041-221 7467 (Tue 7-10 pm).

Northern Ireland

Belfast Aids Helpline, PO Box 44, Belfast BT1 1SH: 0232-226117.

Around Great Britain

Bournemouth Aids Support Group: 0202-38850 (24-hour answering service; staffed Mon & Tue 8-10 pm).

Bradford/West Yorkshire Aids Line: 0274-732939 (Wed & Fri 7.30-9.30 pm).

Brighton Aids Support Line: 0273-74331 (Mon-Fri 8-10 pm).

Bristol Aled Richards Trust: 0272-273436 (Thu 7-9 pm).

Calm: South Coast area, PO Box 11, Bognor Regis, W. Sussex PO21 1AH: 0243-776998 (Mon, Wed, Fri 7.30-10 pm).

Cambridge Aids Helpline, PO Box 257, Cambridge: 0223-69765 (Tue & Wed 7.30-10.30 pm).

Cardiff Aids Helpline, PO Box 304, Cardiff CF2 1YD: 0222-40101/2 (Mon 8-10 pm).

Colchester Aids Helpline: 0206-560225 (Mon-Fri 7-9 pm).

Coventry Aids Helpline: 0203-714144 (Mon 7-10 pm).

Dudley Information Aids Line, c/o Corbett Hospital, Home Wardens' Office, Stourbridge: 0384-390390 ask for Dial (Wed 7-10 pm).

Gwent Aids Helpline: (Caerleon) 0633-422532 (Tue 2-8 pm); (Newport): 0633-841091 (Mon-Fri 8.30 am to 4.30 pm).

Leeds Aids Advice, PO Box HP7, Leeds LS6 1PD: 0532-444209 (Mon & Thur 7-9 pm).

Manchester Aidsline: 061-228 1617 (Mon-Fri 7-10 pm).

Merseyside Aids Helpline: 051-708 0234 (Wed 7-10 pm).

Nottingham Aids Helpline: 0602-585526 (Mon & Tue 7-10 pm).

Oxford, Oxaids: 0865-246036 (Wed 6-8 pm).

Plymouth Aids Support Group: 0752-663609.

Preston Aidsline: 0772-555556 (Mon 7-9.30 pm).

Reading Aidsline, PO Box 75, Reading: 0734-503377 (Thu 8-10 pm).

Sheffield Aids Support Group: 0742-663870 (evenings).

Solent Aids Helpline: 0703-37363 Ansaphone (Tue, Thur, Sat 7.30-10.00 pm).

South Lincolnshire: 0476-60192; 0205-54462 (24-hr answer-phone).

Sussex Aids Helpline, PO Box 17, Brighton: 0273-743316 (Mon-Fri 8-10 pm).

West Midlands Aidsline: 021-6221511 (Tue & Thu 7.30-10.00 pm).

West Sussex/Hampshire: 0243-776998 (Mon, Wed, Fri 7.30-10 pm).

Some other useful numbers

Aids North
PO Box 1BD
Newcastle upon Tyne
NE99 1BD
091-2322855 (Wed & Fri 7-10 pm)

For help and advice for nurses and health-care workers:

Nurses Support Group
53 Mirlees Court
London SE5 9QW

Haemophiliacs requiring more information should contact:

The Haemophilia Society
PO Box 9
16 Trinity Street
London SE1 1DE
01-407 1010 (Mon to Fri 8.30 am to 5.00 pm)

The Terrence Higgins Trust offers a wide range of educational materials (including a leaflet on the chalice and Aids and an information pack), resources and support services for people with Aids, their families and friends.

Support services include Antibody Positive, for those newly diagnosed as HIV-positive, Frontliners, for those with clinically diagnosed Aids or ARC, an interfaith group, and support groups for women with Aids, the families of patients, the partners of patients. The Trust also offers one-to-one counselling and crisis intervention.

Speakers for study days and conferences are available from the Trust. A minimum of two months notice, and preferably longer, should be given.

Terrence Higgins Trust
BM Aids
London WC1 3XX
(please enclose sae when writing for information)
Offices: 01-831 0330
Helpline: 01-833 2971 (Mon to Fri 7-10 pm; weekends 3-10 pm).

190

*The Society of St Paul and
the Daughters of St Paul
at the service of the Church*

> I became the servant of the Church when God made me responsible for delivering God's message to you, the message which was a mystery hidden for generations and centuries and now has been revealed to his saints.
>
> *St Paul to the Church at Colossae*

Since the days when Christ walked among the stones in the desert places of Palestine, the mind of man has devised wonders for the people of the world. Machinery has changed the nature of labour, great roads speed our way to capital cities; in the twinkling of an eye computers calculate matters most intricate—above all, nations can communicate with one another by radio and television and film, by telephone and telex, by newspapers and magazines and books in every language.

How marvellous to be able to use the power of technology to spread to the entire world the healing message of Christ—to take his words, preached in a little country so long ago, to every corner of the Earth!

This was the dream of young James Alberione as he knelt in a lonely vigil of prayer, on New Year's Eve 1900. And from the inspiration of that vigil was to come, in 1914, the Society of St Paul, the religious congregation of priests and brothers who proclaim the Gospel through the media of social communication. In 1915, he founded the Daughters of St Paul—sisters who would dedicate themselves to the same apostolate.

From their early days both the Society of St Paul and the Daughters of St Paul have poured effort and imagination into making their Founder's dream a reality. Working side by side, they communicate the word of Christ as writers, broadcasters, film-makers, television producers, printers and photographers, publishers and journalists, shop-managers and sales-hands. Under Fr Alberione's vigorous leadership, until his death in 1971, the priests, brothers and sisters have taken root in thirty countries all over the world.

In Britain since 1947, the Society of St Paul publishes books under the imprint of St Paul Publications. The Daughters of St Paul offer their service to the Church through their small but distinctive chain of religious Book and Media Centres.

The Church, at the Second Vatican Council, declared that "it is one of her duties to announce the Good News of Salvation also with the help of the media of social communication and to instruct men in their proper use". The Society of St Paul and the Daughters of St Paul have the Church's official mandate to proclaim the Gospel through the media of social communication.

Characteristics of the two religious congregations as expressed in their Constitutions:

Our aim. Sent to proclaim the Truth, we assume in the Church the specific role she entrusts to us, the work of evangelisation with the media of social communication: press, films, radio, television, records—all the inventions which human progress furnishes and the needs and conditions of the times require.

Our religious witness. We dedicate our strength, our person and our time to this mission to which we are committed as community.

Religious consecration through the vows animates and sustains our apostolic activity and makes us completely available for the service of Truth.

Our target. Animated by the spirit of St Paul, we direct the message to all without distinction of culture, class or boundary. Unable to reach all at once, we seek to reach the masses, giving preference to the poor, to those furthest away from the faith.

Following the example of Christ, we proclaim the message of salvation with fidelity and integrity, adapting it to various mentalities and environmental situations, with due respect for the authentic values found in every culture and tradition.

And our future. Proclaiming the Gospel through the media of social communication is nowadays of critical importance. Many adult Christians still need help in becoming mature Christians. Young people, the hope of the Church, cry out for religious experience, for authentic Christian life. Those in search of truth are to be offered the word of God. The Society of St Paul and the Daughters of St Paul have a major role in this programme. They have laid their foundations, but their work needs to develop and diversify—it needs people who are eager to share with others the wealth of their faith.

MARY'S PLACE
IN CHRISTIAN DIALOGUE

Occasional papers of the
Ecumenical Society of
the Blessed Virgin Mary

edited by Alberic Stacpoole

Foreword incorporating a blessing by Pope John Paul II
Preface by Eric Kemp, Mervyn Alexander and
Gordon Wakefield

V. THE PROTESTANT TRADITION
Embodiment of Unmerited Grace — *Eric W. Gritsch*
From Dysfunction to Disbelief — *Donald G. Dawe*
The Virgin Mary in Methodism — *Gordon S. Wakefield*
Mary: An Evangelical Viewpoint — *Keith Weston*

VI. OTHER TRADITIONS: CHRISTIAN AND
NON-CHRISTIAN
The Mother of God in Orthodox Theology and Devotion —
    Kallistos Ware
Mary in Syriac Tradition — *Sebastian Brock*
A Woman in Israel — *Nicholas de Lange*
Mary in Islam — *R. J. McCarthy*

VII. HISTORICAL
The English tradition of the Doctrine of the Immaculate
    Conception — *Alberic Stacpoole*
Cardinal Newman's Teaching about the Blessed Virgin Mary
    — *Charles S. Dessain*
Pope Pius XII and the Blessed Virgin Mary — *H. E. Cardinale*

VIII. DEVOTIONAL
Intercession — *Gordon S. Wakefield*
Living Lourdes — *A. G. C. King*

0 85439 201 7   297 pages   hardbound £10.00

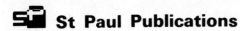 **St Paul Publications**

THE FIRST DAY AFTER THE SABBATH...

I ran to the tomb and... LK 24,1

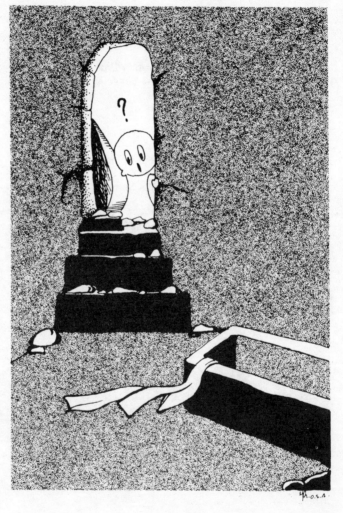

THE GREATEST JOY
OF MY LIFE:

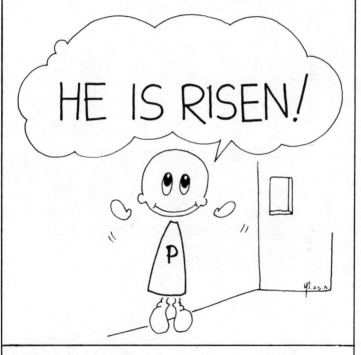

The two illustrations are from *Do you love me?*: a delightful little book on the fascinating adventure of following Jesus and the sweeping message of his teaching. Also in the same series: *Late have I loved you* (on St Augustine) and *One of those who said Yes* (The story of a call). All published by St Paul Publications. £3.25 each.